RSD in Me!

Julie,
Thanks for all of
your help!.
Barby Allyn Ingle

Barby Allyn Ingle-Taylor

Revised: September 5, 2011

RSD in Me!

A Patient And Caretaker Guide To Reflex Sympathetic Dystrophy And Other Chronic Pain Conditions

This book goes through aspects of chronic pain and Reflex Sympathetic Dystrophy/Complex Regional Pain Syndrome (RSD/CRPS) including definition, causes, tips on dealing with healthcare professionals, information for caretakers, emotional aspects of dealing with chronic pain, and tips on coping with the pain. I wrote this book as a pain patient, based on my experiences in dealing with pain and the healthcare system. In 1994, I earned a degree in Social Psychology from George Mason University. I then worked as a head cheer and dance coach at a Division IA University and was a business owner of a successful cheerleading company until my accident in 2002. This book is not intended to take the place of your healthcare professionals or treating doctors.

Author

Barby Allyn Ingle-Taylor

Editor

Ray Bilkie

RSD in Me!

INDEX

SECTION ONE

HOW DO YOU KNOW?

WHY A BOOK ON RSD

In 2002, I was in a minor car accident and diagnosed with whiplash. After months of getting worse and noticing new symptoms, I was diagnosed with a shoulder injury and depression, having many doctors tell me it was all in my head. Many of the tests performed did not show any problems. Even so, my symptoms were still bad and becoming detrimental. I went to see over 35 doctors. One doctor performed a vascular study on me and found a lack of blood flow to my right arm, neck and face. He insisted that I needed surgery right away.

Willing to do anything to get out of pain, I went into the hospital to have my first rib taken out to make room for my nerves and blood flow. I thought that this would fix all my pain, but I was wrong. The surgeon did a poor job with the surgery and I ended up with spurs growing on my stump of a rib and pain much more severe than I had at the start. After five lung collapses, I went to a new surgeon. He did a body scan in 3-D and saw the problem right away. One spur was hooked into my nerve bundle in my shoulder and the other went directly into my right lung. I had surgery a few days later on the rib to remove these spurs.

Since about a month after the accident, I attended physical therapy, which was excruciating and seemed to make things worse. Finally, in May of 2005, I found my way to a pain clinic here in Arizona. My doctor took the time to listen to my history and look at me. The thought of being examined again was frightening. After an hour with me, he said he thought I had Reflex Sympathetic Dystrophy (RSD) and wanted to run yet another test. He told me he was going to stick a needle into my neck and put a chemical of some sort in my ganglion nerve bundle. If the test worked and the pain was helped even for a short time, it meant that I did have RSD, as all my signs and symptoms had pointed to all this time.

The thing is, I had a doctor, four months earlier, tell me that he was 100 percent sure that I did not have RSD. This same doctor did an electromyography (EMG) on me 6 times, which was awful enough, so the thought of a test that involved a needle was beyond scary. I had found a site on the web and put in my symptoms, even the ones that did not seem to fit with the others. After the site led me to www.rsdhope.org, I was sure I had the symptoms. Why didn't my original doctors believe me? They saw the symptoms, saw me walk into walls and pass out from the severe pain and more. When my new doctor, Dr. Mark Rubin, suggested that I might have RSD, my first response was, "Dr. Steier was sure I did not." But what test had Dr. Steier done to be so sure? NOT ONE!

After finding so little information out there and having so many doctors, who did not know about RDS, try to treat me, I realized that I am the one who has to teach my caretakers. While teaching them, I have learned so much myself that I was inspired to write this book and video series because they are tools I wish I had in my starting stages of RSD. I want you to have the whole story. In my research, I have found very little literature that tells the whole story; I know how important it is to have the big picture. What information is out there? What is fact and what is fiction? What is old news and what are the newest options for patients?

Chronic or life-threatening illnesses can have a devastating impact on your entire life. I have come to realize that I am the only one responsible for my health. Many doctors who are not connected with a research hospital or university do not have the time to keep up to the minute with the latest information. RSD is just one type of chronic pain. It does not always respond to treatments that other chronic pain conditions would be regularly helped by, though. Even among RSD patients there are differences in response to treatments, as RSD is a fluid dystrophy.

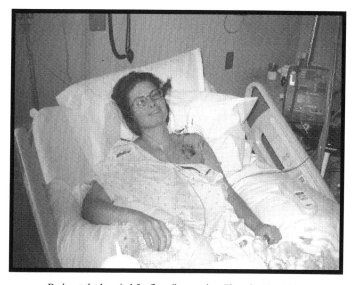

Barby at the hospital for first rib resection, Phoenix, Nov 2003

Sharing this information with you in an easy to understand language has come to be my purpose. If I had a resource like this when I started, I would have spent a lot less time, money and frustration. As I have come to know, RSD does not yet have a cure and only a small number of RSD'ers will ever go into remission. Do not lose hope. There is research going on and the government is taking notice of this debilitating syndrome. This book is intended for RSD patients and caretakers who have a need for more advanced, in-depth medical information and tips for daily living. This information is not always readily available to you or put in terms that are easy to understand. Another goal of this project is to educate patients and their families about their treatment options so that they can better understand, communicate, and make informed decisions about medical treatments, along with the specific needs of the person in their life with RSD.

The book is based on facts I have gathered and myths I have seen exposed along my journey. The video production has involved a team of people who have experienced RSD as patients, family members, caretakers, and doctors. We will cover a diverse range of topics in this production. The team approach for development and production of *RSD in ME!* is designed to ensure accuracy and understanding to make your life better. This book can serve as a starting point for communication between your family, team of doctors and you.

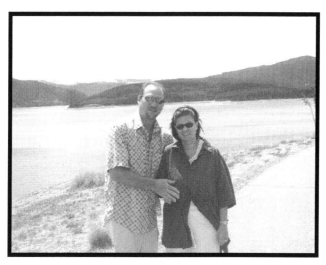

Ken and Barby taking a break from the hospital in Colorado, May 2004

RSD can be a lifelong condition that can have a significant impact not only on the patient but on family and friends as well. The condition affects many aspects of the patient's life in varying degrees. For me, the simple things are the toughest. Daily living activities such as personal grooming, as well as my social and personal life, have all been affected. I lost my professional life to the bad days of RSD, also due to not being prepared for a catastrophic injury. I have had to adjust my daily routine because of the inability and difficulty of performing work-related tasks.

I participate in very limited leisure activities as I had to find my tolerance levels and work within them. I used to be very athletic and loved hiking, biking, and

7

dancing. I constantly worked out and trained. Now I have a limited exercise regimen. Because of my pain, falls and blackouts as well as medication side effects, I am no longer able to drive. I need assistance with shopping, cooking, remembering things and traveling. I am in constant need of help, which makes traveling, social activities, personal care and holidays more complicated. I have difficulty sleeping and experience stress in my daily life. All these combined, as well as financial issues and lack of energy, help the cycle of pain continue. Over time, I have found that pre-planning for daily events, activities and trips is not something I should do out of convenience; it is something I *have to do* to be able to function at even a basic capacity. I created a journal, tracked activities and developed plans to accomplish my goals physically.

Financially, I was wiped out. RSD created a financial strain on my family and me. Because of my lack of income and my medical expenses, RSD has placed an additional burden on everyone in my life. I am lucky to have qualified for social security disability, while many RSD and other chronic pain sufferers have not. Staying on top of my finances and setting out a plan has helped me reduce stress in this area. Getting advice from a tax accountant or financial planner can also reduce stress levels for patients and their families.

Overall, studies show that quality of life for patients of RSD is lower than those with other chronic diseases and chronic pain. People suffering with diabetes, migraines and chronic lung disease all score higher in quality of life studies. Despite this, I find that prayer, having a low stress lifestyle, and hope keeps me in a positive place mentally. I have learned not to sweat the small stuff, to let go of troubles from the past and look for ways to better my future. With a good team around you, the same is possible for you.

RSD is an invisible disability. It is harder to get ahead or be understood when you have an invisible disability. Often times, people have misconceptions about people with disabilities, and some employers may not consider hiring you if they know about your disability. One of the challenging aspects of dealing with my RSD is deciding when, or if, I should disclose it to the people I meet. I choose to disclose my condition to anyone who will listen to let them know that RSD exists and because of the importance of early detection and proper treatment to chances of remission. The more people I educate, the bigger the chances that someone else who has RSD will have it easier. I am strong and am not bothered by the people who believe I might be making it up for attention or other reasons. I know what I live and I want to help others. Not everyone is able to do this. There are some suggestions in later chapters of this book that address when and how to disclose your RSD or other invisible disability.

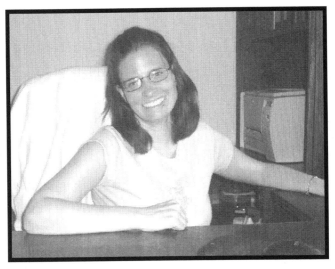

Barby on a Good Day

GENERAL DEFINITION OF RSD

Reflex Sympathetic Dystrophy (RSD) Syndrome does not exist in the absence of pain and usually occurs after an injury takes place. With RSD, your body does not get the message to check the automatic inflammatory response, which occurs at the beginning stages. When the stimulus is no longer present, the pain becomes sympathetically driven. Therefore, even if the original injury should no longer be an issue, the patient experiences major pain. We all know this condition as Reflex Sympathetic Dystrophy Syndrome (RSD) or Complex Regional Pain Syndrome (CRPS). Doctors and researchers are not exactly sure why the Sympathetic Nervous System (SNS) malfunctions. When the SNS continues the healing process even after the stimulus is gone, it causes continuous severe pain and tissue destruction.

The SNS kicking into action is the body's natural reaction to heal an injury. Generally, to heal, the body must go through a series of events to ensure proper healing of an injury. This starts with the body's inflammatory response. Just as your body sends out healing cells to fight an infection when you're sick, your injury stimulates its own healing medication to "fix" the injury. This process usually takes place within minutes or hours following the injury.

Symptoms and signs of RSD vary from patient to patient, but all of us feel pain. Pain is the one common aspect for us, yet it is hard to understand. Usually RSD develops after a minor injury or trauma. This can be a sprained ankle, a prick from a hypodermic needle, surgical wounds, or, in my case, whiplash injuries exacerbated by additional surgeries. The pain is so out of balance with the original injury that others begin to believe it is all "in our heads." Luckily, there is research going on to help us all understand that this is a real syndrome and a problem that needs attention and solutions for millions of RSD'ers. Many uninformed people, such as medical professionals, therapists, family and friends, believe our symptoms are caused by a psychological disorder. The fact is our general health is seriously affected with RSD. The deep burning sensation becomes so sensitive that touching something, or someone touching you, can cause pain that seems to be from nothing.

RECAP

- Doctors and researchers are not sure why exactly the Sympathetic Nervous System malfunctions.

- Symptoms and signs of RSD vary from patient to patient, but all of us feel pain.

- Usually RSD develops after a minor injury or trauma.

- The deep burning sensation becomes so sensitive that touching something or someone touching you causes pain that seems to be from nothing.

- The feeling of misunderstanding and mistrust from others is one cause of our psychological issues, not the other way around.

RSD HISTORY

RSD has been documented since the Civil War under many different names. It was first studied by Dr. Weir Mitchell. In October of 1864, Dr. Mitchell and his associates, G.R. Moorheouse and W.W. Keen, published a book called *"Gunshot Wounds and Other Injuries of Nerves."* This book reveals some of the symptoms and signs first observed at Turners Alne Hospital for Nervous Diseases in Philadelphia. The description is so much like RSD that it will stick in your mind, and, if you are the patient, it will sound familiar to what you are currently feeling.

"In our early experience of nerve wounds, we met with a small number of men [who] were suffering from a pain which they described as 'burning' or as 'mustard red-hot' or as 'red-hot file rasping the skin'. The seat of burning pain is very various; but it never attacks the trunk, rarely the arm or thigh, and not often the forearm and leg." [1] Since this statement, we have found that RSD can affect the trunk, arms, legs, and internal organs. RSD can be body wide or in one or more extremities. For example, I have

---

[1] Gunshot Wounds and Other Injuries of Nerves, Mitchell, Moorheouse, Keen, 1864.

RSD in my face, neck, shoulder, arm, hand and foot. RSD was first described in the 19th century with severe chronic pain and other symptoms such as swelling, excessive sweating, and changes in skin color and temperature. The same collection of symptoms that were true to RSD in the 19th century is a part of the condition today. Modern science has also added new symptoms to the list with better understanding and research over the years.

Mitchell's description of burning pain and red-hot file rasping the skin are words RSD patients still connect with today. Mitchell first used the term Causalgia, which means "the burning pain," when describing his patients' symptoms. It was right on the money then and still is today. We must now teach doctors to see the signs sooner. A diagnosis, treatment and understanding should be quickly and aggressively pursued for better chances of remission. My understanding from speaking with healthcare professionals is that RSD is not taught in medical school as a requirement and when it is taught, less than half a day is spent on it. Unless a doctor, nurse, EMT or other healthcare professional is interested in pursuing more information, the likelihood of them being able to spot, diagnose and treat their patients becomes slim.

Since Mitchell named this condition Causalgia, there have been over twenty name designations. Some of them include: Algodystrophy, Sudeck's Atrophy, Regional Pain Syndrome, Complex Regional Pain Syndrome (CRPS), Reflex Sympathetic Dystrophy (RSD), Post Traumatic Dystrophy, Painful Post-Traumatic Dystrophy, Painful Post-Traumatic Osteoporosis, and Transient Migratory Osteoporosis. No matter the name, RSD is the worst pain condition known to man, and those of us with it would agree totally. According to the McGill pain scale, a rating system used internationally to measure pain, RSD rates worse than cancer, childbirth with no medications, amputation, and all others on the list.

In the early 1920's German physicians began a focus on RSD, then referring to it as Causalgia. A greater understanding came during and after WWI. Researcher Athanassio-Benisty described movement disorders such as tremors relating to Causalgia. Both Athanassio-Benisty and Tinel detailed peripheral nerve injuries and Causalgia and a possible connection to a sympathetic origin. Other doctors provided additional research on symptoms of RSD such as glossy skin, skin temperature changes and reflex involvement. Some later doctors such as Purves-Stewart,

Evans and Carter used Mitchell as a reference when working on research and patients. Mitchell's findings were also the basis of research by French doctors to further finding the origin of RSD. Although German physicians described Causalgia, they did not use the term, and this may be because Mitchell's findings were not translated into German. In all, RSD has been studied around the world by many researchers, scientists and physicians. They have come to many of the same conclusions as to the symptoms that RSD causes for many.[2]

---

[2] J Hist Neurosci. Journal of the History of Neurosciences, 2004 Dec, 13 (4):326-35.

RECAP

- RSD has been documented since the Civil War under many different names.

- In October of 1864, Weir Mitchell and his associates, G.R. Moorheouse and W.W. Keen, published a book called *"Gunshot Wounds and Other Injuries of Nerves"*.

- A few years later, Mitchell first used the term Causalgia (the burning pain).

- We must now teach doctors to see the signs sooner so that a diagnosis, treatment and understanding are quickly and aggressively pursued.

CAUSES OF RSD

Although a lot of research is being done, we are still not sure exactly what causes RSD. A history of trauma as a possible cause is found in most research. The most common thought is that RSD is caused by minor injuries or surgical procedures. In ¼ of RSD patients, there is no cause that can be identified. The injury was so minor or occurred long before the pain became disabling that the patient just cannot remember what minor trauma may have caused RSD to develop. Doctors do not all agree, but there is some possible speculation about where the pain starts turning into RSD. There are two types of processes with the pain of RSD: sympathetically maintained pain (SMP) and sympathetically independent pain (SIP). The good news is that RSD patients with SMP can experience improvement or relief of RSD pain with therapy directed at the sympathetic nervous system (SNS). For those with SIP, it is not as easy, but it is still possible to find relief. SIP is associated with the central nervous system, which is thought to involve the organs and therefore is less responsive to pain treatments.

There has been some progress on finding causes of RSD. However, we still do not know why some people develop this horrible syndrome and others heal with no problems. RSD is not known to be hereditary. The typical cause is a specific event, which sometimes is so insignificant that you may not remember it occurring.

These events can be:

- A spider bite
- Cardiovascular events or conditions
- Immobilization from a fracture or sprain
- Injury to the affected limb
- Neoplasm- tumor or tissue containing a growth
- Neurological events or conditions
- Surgical procedures such as carpal tunnel, knee arthroscopy, hip arthroplasty
- Trauma- Minor or Major

For me, after the accident, the injury to my brachial plexus was considered the issue and for a long period, no effort was made to look for other conditions such as RSD. Upper extremity RSD may be missed because of a brachial plexus injury that gradually develops into SMP and then

20

into RSD. Some doctors may also see RSD as part of neurological conditions, such as carpal tunnel syndrome or pinched spinal nerves. In addition, certain types of cancers may produce RSD-like symptoms, and those with heart problems or stroke have been reported as risk factors for developing RSD.

Before you can be diagnosed with RSD, your doctor needs to eliminate the possibility for other causes of RSD-like symptoms. These have to be considered and ruled out before a definite diagnosis of RSD can be established. For instance, some other reasons for RSD-like symptoms are:

- Bursitis
- Cancers
- Cellulites
- Diabetic Neuropathy
- Femoral/Tibia Injury Or Fracture
- Gout
- Lumbar or Cervical Disk Hernia
- Lymphedema
- Meniscus Tears
- Nerve Entrapment Syndromes (e.g., Carpal Tunnel Syndrome)

- Osteomyelitis (Bone Infection)
- Patella (Kneecap) Injuries
- Peripheral Neuropathy
- Rheumatoid Arthritis
- Septic Arthritis
- Shoulder Injuries
- Tendonitis
- Thoracic Outlet Syndrome
- TMJ
- Vascular Insufficiency

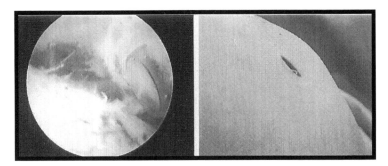

Barby during should surgery May 2003

SYMPTOMS: PAIN + A WHOLE LOT MORE

The symptoms of RSD vary from patient to patient. Remember, as discussed earlier, the only symptom that every RSD'er has is severe pain. If the patient has not been properly diagnosed yet, these symptoms can cause extreme duress and confusion to all involved. There are four main categories for our symptoms. The categories are constant chronic burning pain, emotional disturbances, inflammation, and spasms in blood vessels and muscles of the extremities. You should have at least one symptom in three of the four categories to be diagnosed with RSD.

These categories have their own symptoms associated with them. Symptoms include pain, swelling, sweating, spasms, emotional disturbances, short-term memory problems, sleep disorder, and other medical issues. Effects of RSD can be reversed to give patients a better chance at remission. As the RSD takes over, we tend to have a personality change. We grow irritable, anxious; our suffering is evident in our actions and changing expressions. Sleeping becomes a problem. For many of us, being in one position for too long increases the pain levels.

We are often barred from sleep by severe, sharp and burning pain. I also experience a feeling of electric shock, which can come at any time. I have dropped many plates, drinks and anything I was trying to hold onto from these sudden shocks. As I lose sleep, I also have an increase in hypersensitivity. The heightened sensitivity causes simple things such as a breeze, light or a loud noise to increase the pain. These drastic symptoms are usually caused by a minor injury, which is one of the hardest things to comprehend about RSD.

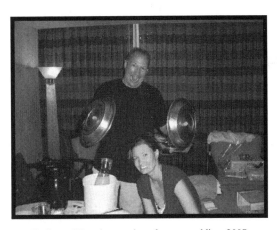

Barby and Ken the morning after our wedding, 2007

- Pain
  - "Aching, burning, crushing, dull, electric, feeling as if you're on fire, sharp, stabbing, throbbing, tingling" are some ways to describe the pain.
  - The pain can be anywhere around the affected area, not always right on the site of the trauma.
  - The affected area is usually hot or cold to the touch.
  - The pain will be more severe than expected for the type of injury sustained.
  - The affected area has a lowered threshold to pain from external stimuli.
  - Extreme sensitivity to touch: something as simple as a slight touch, clothing, sheets, even a breeze across the skin on the affected area can cause extreme pain to the patient
  - Sounds and vibrations, especially sharp sudden sounds and deep vibrations, can also increase pain.
  - The softest touch can now cause pain instead of pleasure.

25

- Sweating
  - An increase usually occurs
- Spasms
  - The spasms can be confined to one area or be rolling in nature; moving up and down the leg, arm, or back.
  - Body fatigue
  - Coldness in the affected extremity
- Dystonia
  - Tremors
  - Muscle cramps
- Swelling
  - It takes various forms: the skin may appear mottled, become easily bruised, or have a shiny, dry, red, and tight look to it.
  - Swelling is not always present.
  - Swelling can spread to involve a larger area and becomes brawny (hard).
- Muscle and skin tightness
  - Edema - swelling that is usually localized to the affected limb and may have a well demarcated edge.

- Emotional Disturbances
  - Depression
  - RSD causes depression, NOT the other way around
  - Agitation
  - Irritability

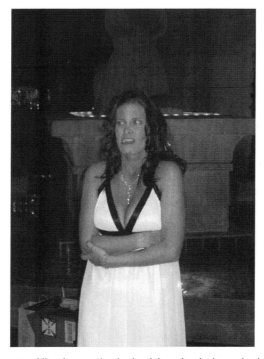

Barby on my wedding day experiencing breakthrough pain, increasing irritability

- Short-term memory problems
  - It becomes easy to lose track of things like whether you took your pills or what you were just talking about.
  - Loss of short-term memory is a part of RSD.
  - Many patients think they are losing their mind as their ability to remember things greatly decreases, but you are NOT losing your mind.
  - Other signs of problems here would include the inability to think of, um, well, ah, hmm, just the right word.
  - The patient's ability to concentrate is also lessened while their irritability is increased.
  - These problems get even worse as the sleep deprivation cycle continues.

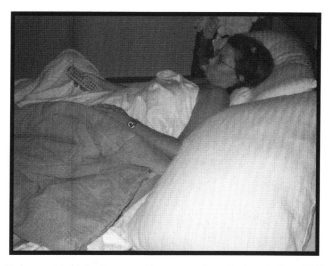

Barby was not able to sleep normal hours, sometimes for days at a time, 2004

- Sleep Disorder/Insomnia

  - Insomnia is often experienced.

  - Disrupted sleep pattern

  - Inability to let the body drift into rapid eye movement (REM) sleep

  - REM sleep allows the body to use its own healing abilities. Without it, the patient's pain cycle continues and becomes more entrenched.

  - As the body cannot heal itself, it becomes harder to achieve REM sleep, which makes the pain worse and so, the cycle continues.

- Other Possible Symptoms
  - Limbic system of the brain
    - Causes many problems that may not be linked to a disease like RSD at first
  - Bone Changes
    - Softening of the bones, Osteoarthritis, Osteoporosis, joint stiffness/ tenderness
    - Thinning and weakness of your bones become more evident
    - At risk for more fractures
  - Nails/Hair
    - On affected extremity, they may grow at a faster/slower rate or become grooved and brittle
    - Hair may become coarse and may be followed by hair loss
  - Color/Skin Changes
    - Skin may turn shiny, red, dry and tightened
    - Skin may atrophy
  - General Weakness/ Movement Disorders
    - Increased body fatigue, fever, rashes, sores

- Difficulty in beginning or general movement of the injured part
  - Joint stiffness resulting in limited range of motion
  - Increased reflex reactions
  - Balance/Coordination
- Miscellaneous
  - Dizziness
  - Horner's syndrome
  - Increased muscle tone
  - Low-grade fever
  - Permanent damage to muscles and joints
  - Tinnitus
  - Visual disturbances such as blurriness, dry eyes, and others

GETTING DIAGNOSED THE RIGHT WAY

The importance of a prompt diagnosis is that early treatment is equivalent to higher chances of remission or a lowering of symptoms, in comparison to a later treatment. In my experience, many doctors either have never heard of or do not know all they should about RSD. Many will run tests such as MRI, MRA, X-Rays, EMG, heart tests, vision, hearing, and so on. I even had a dentist tell me I have TMJ based on the pain in the right side of my face. As discussed previously, the likelihood of any other underlying medical condition that could cause the level of pain or dysfunction being experienced by the patient must be ruled out. These issues lead to delayed diagnosis and fewer chances to correct or put the RSD into remission. Earlier diagnosis will lead to better treatment options, preserve mobility, prevent emotional issues and help deal with this nasty syndrome.

There are two types of Reflex Sympathetic Dystrophy. RSD Type I is when the syndrome is caused by a simple injury. Examples of simple injuries include whiplash, sprain or strain, athletics, falling over, needle poke, broken bone, or a minor operation. The simple injury is what causes a nerve or tissue to get injured and the resulting pain is totally disproportionate to the injury. A severe, intense burning pain that is not relieved by strong painkillers marks it. If not treated in a timely manner, the pain may go on years after the initial injury has healed. RSD Type II has the same clinical features as RSD Type I except for the presence of clinical signs and history consistent with a nerve injury.[3] With RSD Type II, there is no apparent injury to incite the syndrome. According to the International Association for the Study of Pain criteria, the characteristic features required to establish the diagnosis of RSD Type I are as follows: (1) the presence of an initiating noxious event or a cause of immobilization; (2) continuing pain, Allodynia, or Hyperalgesia with pain disproportionate to any inciting event; (3) evidence at some time of edema, changes in skin blood flow, or abnormal Sudomotor activity in the region of the pain; and (4) the exclusion of medical conditions that would otherwise account for the degree of pain and dysfunction. Motor disturbances and

---

[3] Anesthesiology: May 2002 - Volume 96 - Issue 5 - pp 1254-1260, Clinical Concepts and Commentary, Complex Regional Pain Syndrome I (Reflex Sympathetic Dystrophy), Raja, Srinivasa N. M.D.; Grabow, Theodore S. M.D.

atrophic changes, such as altered nail and hair growth may be observed in some cases.

Until a few years ago, there was no way to test for or confirm RSD. Far too often, patients are not believed because there is no way objectively to measure pain. New information has become available and hopes for a possible single test are on the horizon. Currently, there is no single test for RSD. Every patient must be diagnosed by the physician based on the patient's history, physical examination, tests to rule out other causes and more tests for changes in pathology. More research needs to be done, but these guidelines are a step in the right direction.

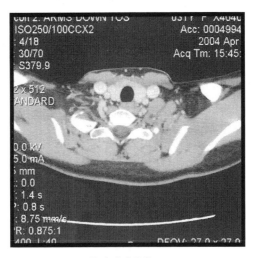

Barby's 3-D Scan

Professionals on a regularly basis are now using a few tests and procedures that are appropriate for diagnosing RSD. These tests include: Thermogram, ganglion nerve block, small nerve biopsy, and a patient's clinical history (signs and symptoms). In addition, X-rays can show thinning of bones (osteoporosis), and Functional MRI Nuclear Bone Scans can show characteristic uptake patterns. These help diagnose RSD. Unfortunately, there is no specific blood test or other single diagnostic test that can confirm a RSD diagnosis.

The test used to find out if I had RSD was the sympathetic nerve block (SNB). There are some advantages to this procedure as a test for RSD. If you are positive for RSD in your upper extremity, after administering the SNB, you will have almost instant relief. However, the drawbacks are that the relief does not last, and you may still be positive for RSD, even if no relief was apparent.

TECHNICALLY, WHAT IS RSD?

RSD is believed to represent an exaggerated response of the sympathetic nervous system to some form of injury. Unlike a normal recovery from an injury or trauma, RSD results in chronic irritation and pain. The sympathetic nervous system (SNS) along with the parasympathetic nervous system comprises the autonomic nervous system.

The motor neurons of the SNS originate in the spinal cord and run parallel to the spinal cord on both sides. The SNS regulates involuntary responses to stress, such as increased heart rate and constriction of peripheral blood vessels. The nerve fibers leave the spinal cord and are distributed to the heart, lungs, intestines, blood vessels and sweat glands. Research indicates that the SNS also has a role in neuropathic and inflammatory pain. In patients with RSD, there may be evidence of impairment of the SNS function, which is not necessarily limited to the affected extremity.[4]

---

[4] Etiology of Pain in Reflex Sympathetic Dystrophy, medifocushealth.com

The theory is that pain in RSD is caused by an exaggerated response of the SNS to some form of insult or injury to the body. The idea is encouraged by the clinical observation of a nerve block. The nerve block procedure is used to affect the SNS. The sympathetic block procedure results in immediate relief of pain in some RSD patients. For me, it lasts for about two to three hours. For some others, I have heard that it does nothing for them.

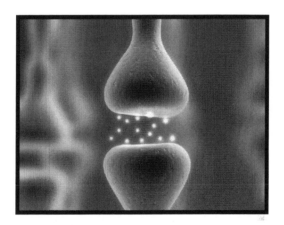

The term Reflex Sympathetic Dystrophy is considered somewhat misleading since only a subset of patients respond to sympathetic blocks indicating that not all pain in this syndrome is related to sympathetically based pain. In addition, dystrophy is only present in a subset of patients and there is little evidence of a reflex mechanism in many patients. In response to these inconsistencies, the International Association for the Study of Pain (IASP) adopted the term Complex Regional Pain Syndrome (CRPS) in 1994 to also describe the debilitating pain syndrome that develops after a relatively minor injury to an extremity (arm or leg), but lasts longer than the actual injury and is more severe than would otherwise be expected from such an injury.[5] It is important to keep in mind that not all patients have the same symptoms, nor do they respond to the same treatments to help relieve their pain. RSD is fluid in nature, meaning physical symptoms will come and go.

---

[5] International Association for the Study of Pain (IASP)

RECAP

- RSD is believed to represent an exaggerated response of the sympathetic nervous system to some form of injury.

- The sympathetic nervous system (SNS) along with the parasympathetic nervous system comprises the autonomic nervous system.

- Research indicates that the SNS also has a role in neuropathic and inflammatory pain.

- Pain in RSD is believed to be caused by an exaggerated response of the SNS.

- The International Association for the Study of Pain (IASP) adopted the term Complex Regional Pain Syndrome (CRPS) in 1994 to also describe the debilitating pain syndrome RSD.

BELIEVING RSD IS REAL

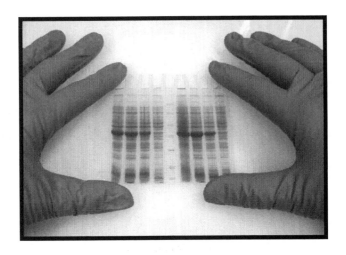

One of my greatest frustrations has been the lack of an explanation for the symptoms of RSD and why it starts in the first place. Recently, a study by co-authors Julia Rissmiller; Lisa Gelman; Li Zheng, MD, PhD; Yuchiao Chang, PhD; and Ralph Gott, all from the Massachusetts General Hospital, has identified a cause of RSD. This takes RSD out of the realm of "it is all in your head" or an emotional disturbance. As I quickly found out, many people are skeptical and some physicians are reluctant to treat you. Doctors sometimes see RSD patients as complainers or malingerers. The willingness to show any sensitivity is lacking from these doctors and caretakers. If you find yourself with a doctor like this, I suggest you get a new doctor, but do not give up on finding some relief for your RSD. For our families, doctors, and our own peace of mind, we need to focus on why the same injuries cause long-term problems in some patients but not in others. This may help lead to a better way of diagnosing RSD, create new treatments and help support groups and family members comprehend the changes that are occurring.

In September '07, Dr Robert Schwartzman addressed the members of the American Association of Pain Management as the keynote speaker. He started by saying, "I finally have something to report."[6] He reported his findings and documentation on how RSD works at a biochemical level, how it affects us inside our brains (as a result of RSD development, not the other way around), and that because now that we know how it develops, we can find a cure. There is hope for us. RSD is fully reversible and, according to Dr. Schwartzman, "We just have to find the way to reverse it." Effects of RSD can be reversed, plus patients have better chances of recovery and remission.

---

[6] Dr. Robert Schwartzman, Keynote speaker for the American Association of Pain Management conference in Las Vegas, Sept 2007

HOW RSD IS PERCEIVED BY THE PATIENT

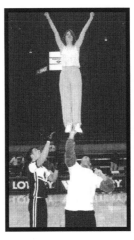

Barby in a cheerleading stunt after a home basketball game in 2001

After college, I had built a great life with my husband for ten years. I got to live out all of my dreams and start making new ones. Although my marriage started having trouble the year prior to the RSD, I was dedicated to making my marriage work. When I became so debilitated by the pain and doctors could not figure out what was going on, I could no longer hold my life together. When my symptoms first began, I thought I was being ridiculous. First, I lost my dream job: coaching cheer and dance at a division I-A University. My business started to crumble and eventually closed. My marriage fell apart and my husband stopped supporting me completely. He actually had me feeling that it was all in my head and tried to convince my family and our friends of the same. The only thing was that I knew was that I would not do this to myself. I began marriage counseling a few months before the accident because of our struggling relationship. After the accident, I continued with counseling for six months and then have went off and on after I found out that this RSD was permanent. Did I have something wrong with me physically? Was it in my head? With more pain, vision difficulties, doctors, blackouts, memory trouble and so on, the worse my life became. I began taking depression and anxiety medication on a regular basis. I really did not know what to think anymore; who was I? I asked everyone around me what they thought I should do. I no longer trusted what my body was telling me. I tried to convince myself that things were in my head and that I was strong enough to get over the pain and other symptoms on my own. I thought I just needed to try harder. I constantly questioned my actions and stopped trusting my instincts. Through counseling, I got my voice back, renewed my confidence, found who I am, and what I am made of. This all helped me face the fact that this pain is a new reality for me, but I was going to find a way to LIVE. I went to a compassionate doctor, Dr. French, in Washington State, which was where I was living at the time. After he did his poking and prodding on me, he diagnosed me with a brachia plexus shoulder injury. It was then recommended to me to get doctors that were more specialized.

Some of my healthcare professionals in Washington found a doctor and physical therapist in Arizona that specialized in athletic injuries. Since I was an athlete, this made sense to me. This Arizona doctor would help me get back to the athletic state I was at physically prior to the accident. Thinking that it was a good idea, and after losing my job and barely hanging onto my marriage, we packed up and moved to Arizona. The day I arrived in AZ, I started physical therapy. A month later, I was going into surgery to fix my shoulder and finally stop the pain. Even though the MRI and X-rays showed there was no injury, the doctor thought it would be best to go through with the surgery. At that point, I was ready for anything that would stop the pain. After surgery, the pain was not gone, and symptoms became worse. I realized that there is more than one type of physical pain and I was experiencing many of them at the same time. I continued to see more doctors; they were ruling out everything but could not tell me what was wrong.

Finally, I found a neurologist who had some new tests for me to undergo. They came back showing that I now had Thoracic Outlet Syndrome (TOS) and that there was a way to fix it. It would just be one more surgery by a vascular surgeon. The vascular surgeon performed his own vascular study/tests and confirmed the diagnosis. A week later, I was having my first rib removed. This surgery was a lot more complicated and had many risks. At this point, I was separated from my husband and did not know anyone in Arizona to help me except doctors. I began paying a neighbor to drive me to appointments and assist me with daily activities around my house.

Putting my trust in this new person, the only person willing to take care of me (though for a price), I decided to go through with the surgery. This surgery was going to be my miracle. After the surgery, I tried to convince myself that I was all better. And some things were better; I was not so tired. But overall, I was worse off than before, and with new symptoms, life became much harder. I thought the original pain was bad, but at that point, I thought if I had to have pain, I wanted the first pain back. On top of the pain, I now had a problem with my right lung. After five lung collapses, some requiring hospital stays, as well as an additional emergency lung procedure, I was turned over to new doctors who checked out my lung and could not understand why I was developing pneumothoraces.

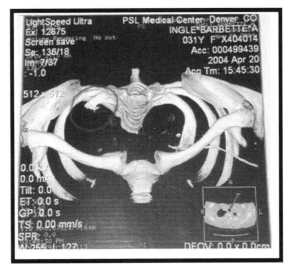

A picture from the 3-D body scan of patient Barby Ingle shows the two spurs on the right first rib after removal. One spur went into the right lung and the other was hooked into the right Brachia Nerve Bundle. The spurs resulted in the need for a repeat of the right first rib resection surgery.

After two months, I went back to the neurologist. My symptoms were worse, and I passed out in his office while he was touching, poking, pulling and examining me.

He realized that there was still a major problem and sent me to a doctor in Colorado. Dr. Brantigan was also a vascular surgeon, but he was one of the doctors who had perfected the TOS surgery. He ran a 3-D body scan and found that the first vascular doctor did a poor job. I had bone spurs, one going into my lung and one going into my nerve bundle. No wonder things were getting worse. I already had a pain in my nerves and the TOS surgery just increased the problem. So, my hope was raised once again. I was going to get one more surgery and be back to my old life.

By this time, I was devastated financially and could no longer pay my neighbor. Luckily, he was intrigued with something he saw in me. He also thought, "Anytime now, she is going to be fine." He moved in with me to take care of me full time. Since I could not pay him, this worked out perfectly. Spending so much time with the only person in AZ I knew who was not a doctor or lawyer, I began to have feelings for him, and we began to date, if you can call it that. I did not get out much.

After this latest surgery, I went into physical therapy again. I had a new PT, and he treated me as if I was a healthy athlete and pushed me through our sessions.

EVERY session, I would leave in severe pain, crying, dizzy, walking into walls and to the point of vomiting. He said he was waiting for me to have a breakthrough. He told me my nerve was stuck and to just keep pushing with the weights and one day it would just pop free! I was getting worse and my drill sergeant of a physical therapist was making it worse. He also could not understand how, although I was hurting so badly, I would not put ice on after my sessions. That would have just been adding insult to my injuries. The ice was excruciating. I had a knee surgery in 2001 where I used ice after surgery to keep the swelling down and I loved it. However, this time the ice was bad, but I did not know why since it worked so well with my knee in the past.

One day, my PT was out of town on business. I was very scared but went with a different therapist from the same office for the week. For once, I was in good hands. Paul, my substitute PT, began by asking me questions. He asked me things about my everyday life (activities of daily living), my symptoms and said he wanted to try a different approach. I was scared but wanted to do anything to get better. He took away all of the weights and machines and began traction and a bit of nerve stretching. The traction was the greatest thing I had experienced in a long time, but the nerve stretching was still excruciating.

Each time he stretched me, he went right back to the traction, which brought the pain level down. This was great; I was finally able to get my arm into a semi-straight position. This was relief from the curled-up limb I was used to by then. I worked with Paul for five months and never went back to my old PT. Paul's specialty was treating patients with chronic pain such as TOS and RSD. We would talk about the symptoms of RSD. I began to look into it on my own through the Internet. So many people were in the same situation as I was, going from doctor to doctor with little to no relief, having a weird collection of symptoms that did not make sense to any of the doctors who saw them.

When I went back to my neurologist for a checkup, I brought what I had printed off of the Internet about RSD and pointed out to him that I thought I had this horrible condition. He assured me that I did not have RSD, and he was 100 percent sure. He decided to send me to a pain specialist to get a shot of cortisone, also known as a trigger point injection.

After all this time, I had finally found him: the doctor who knew. The pain specialist seemed as knowledgeable as Paul and was caring and willing to help. Dr. Rubin listened to me, evaluated me and then put everything together. He thought I might have RSD. He wanted to run a test and it involved a needle. At this point, after going through more EMGs than was reasonable for medical treatment, I was reluctant. I also pointed out that my previous doctor said he was 100 percent sure that I did not have RSD. Dr. Rubin asked me what test my last doctor had performed to determine this. I told him the list of test and surgeries that I had been through over the past 2.5 years. He explained that none of those tests would show RSD and that this test wouldn't be pleasant but would help if I did have RSD. I placed my trust and pain in his hands.

A week later, I had the test. I did not expect any relief. A miracle happened; within 15 minutes of the procedure, I was able to straighten my arm. Although not all the way, it was more than I had in years at this point. Dr. Rubin confirmed the diagnosis of RSD. I had some relief from my pain for the first time since the accident and I had an answer. Although the pain was not completely gone, it was only a four on the pain scale versus the usual ten. This lasted for almost three hours and then the pain returned. It hit me so hard that it was like I had to adjust to the pain level of a nine through ten all over again. On my next visit, he told me about how he could do a procedure called pulsed radiofrequency ablation (PRF). It was a similar setup, but the relief could last weeks, months, and even years. I was skeptical, but if I could just have a few more hours of relief again, it would be worth it. Since then, Dr. Rubin and Paul, my physical therapist, are working out of the same office and are giving me the best treatment I could ask for. One day there may be a cure, but for now, I will take the relief they offer me.

The relief... After the PRF, I became sick, stiff-necked, and feverish for days. I thought that this treatment did not work for me, as many treatments do not work on all RSD patients. Then I began to notice that I did have some relief. It lasted 23 days, and then the pain returned. When I went back in order to see Dr. Rubin we knew this was a promising treatment option for me. Since then, I have had similar results almost every time. Every four to six weeks I receive the PRF and have great success after a few days of bad side effects each time.

At one point, Dr. Rubin wanted to try a full-blown RF procedure instead of the pulsed. We thought that the relief might be greater and went for it. Unfortunately, the few days of horrible side effects turned into three weeks. I went back to him and asked for another procedure after only three weeks. He thought that might be too soon, but it was worth a try. He went back to the PRF and it worked! For some people with RSD this form of treatment only lasts for up to six procedures. I am now past 25 and still getting relief. Dr. Rubin has agreed to perform the procedure on me as often as I needed. Our hope is that one of these future treatments will be the one that last years for me. Until then, I thank God that He brought me to Dr. Rubin and that Dr. Rubin was informed and knowledgeable in RSD. He helps RSD and chronic pain patients, as well as me, to lead lives that are more enjoyable. With Dr. Rubin, we are treated like people who just happen to have RSD. He does not allow me to fall into the trap of RSD becoming me; it is just something in me. Finding a doctor like Dr. Rubin in your area is so important. Do not settle for less! You do not have to!

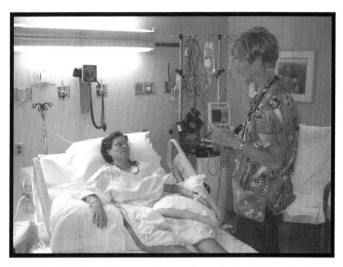

2004- St. Luke's Hospital, Denver Co; second try at the 1st Rib resection Surgery

In September 2007, I was able to attend an American Association for Pain Management (AAPM) meeting for healthcare workers. At this event, Dr. Schwartzman, a leading specialist of RSD in the United States and internationally, presented the Keynote speech. He spoke about Ketamine infusions becoming the most common future treatment for all RSD patients. After his keynote speech, I had the opportunity to speak to him privately for over 30 minutes. We spoke about my story, what I was doing for treatments, and if there was a possibility that it could be affecting me in a negative way over the long term. His opinion was that it was not going to

53

have a negative impact and, if it was working, to keep going until I could get in to see him. I know RSD patients who have been treated by him with Lidocaine and Ketamine infusions who had great success. I asked him if he would be willing to have me as a patient. He told me to call his office and make an appointment. So, I did.

The earliest date I could get was almost two years later. I think Dr. Rubin and his staff here in Phoenix, Arizona is incredible, but they do not offer the Ketamine infusion. Ketamine infusion is a non-invasive procedure that has shown great potential and promise for remission with RSD patients. I cannot pass up this opportunity but am very fortunate that I have a place to turn to if the Ketamine treatment does not work. My doctors here in AZ are all pulling for me. Although I will not get my life back, I am proud of my accomplishments and am happy that I got to live out my dreams before RSD. I now look forward to the day that I can live a more normal life: to work, drive and socialize again. I will have to constantly be careful of new injuries, but I will physically be able to progress in life.

SECTION TWO

WHAT'S NEXT?

WHEN DOES THE PAIN END?

At this point, there is no cure, only remission. Very few RSD patients ever go into remission, but it is possible. In the meantime, you can do some things to make life more enjoyable and bearable. Start by finding the right doctor, test out the pain medicines and procedures that you are comfortable with, and communicate with your doctors, caretakers and family to create a treatment plan that works for you.

I found that the people who were your friends before RSD tend to not handle the thought of you never getting better very well. Lose the people in your life who are not supporting you, whether that person is a doctor or a friend since first grade; you do not need their stress. Your emotional well-being is just as important as finding relief from the pain. I keep track, in a journal, of when pain is stronger, of when symptoms flare, and of general life experiences. I find this helpful in making sure that I am getting the right treatment and that I am not making myself worse.

Remember, for some, the medications you need to take do not have to be of a strong dosage; take what you need for maximum relief and life function. I am using the method of taking the minimum so that I do not build up a tolerance too quickly. Since there is no cure for RSD yet, I want to stretch out what I do have available for relief. After working and communicating with other RSD patients who have had RSD for at least ten years more than me, I see that it can get worse; it can spread, and it can be more pain than you have today, if you can imagine that. Getting the word out, educating people and lobbying for additional research and awareness is our best hope of ending the pain.

When looking for the right doctor to work with you, one who is willing to work with you to treat the RSD in you, ask the important questions. Are there any doctors in my area who specialize in managing RSD patients? You can check with local RSD support groups and also ask the doctors if they have a RSD patient that they are currently treating or have treated in the past so you can speak with them. There are activities you can be doing on your own. You can improve your condition or at least prevent it from getting worse. Keep in mind that with RSD, pain equals no gain. You should not take an athletic mentality or approach to dealing with your RSD. Ask your current/potential doctor, how much experience they have had treating patients with RSD. Does that doctor feel there is one treatment that is better than others or that they are more comfortable performing?

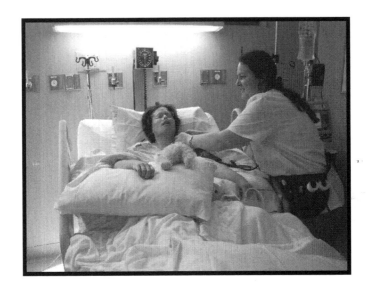

In choosing treatments, I have run into situations with insurance companies where they do not cover the treatment I wish to have. My husband's company seems to change insurers each year, and every insurer has covered different things or needed the treatments coded in a specific way so that they will cover it. It is a good idea to find out what your health insurance policy will cover before treatment is administered.

Every patient is different and responds differently with treatments. Find out what the doctor thinks your short term and long-term prognosis looks like. Create a team of health care professionals. Find out what types of healthcare professionals your doctor thinks should be involved in your treatment. When a treatment is suggested, find out why. What are the pros and cons to the recommendation?

Remember, be the Chief of Staff of your medical team. You are in charge of you, and it is your responsibility to investigate from multiple sources before making a treatment decision that may affect your future. Just because something takes the pain away today does not make it the best option for your future. Ask if the side effects can be reversed and if there are chances of any lasting negative complications prior to any invasive procedure.

RECAP

- Find the right doctor for you.

- Test out the pain medicines. If they don't work for you, stop them and ask for something else.

- Communicate with your doctors, family and caretakers to create a treatment plan.

- Lose the people in your life who are not supporting you.

- Keep a journal to track symptoms, treatments and for your personal well-being.

TREATMENT PLANS

There is no cure for RSD, but progress is being made to find the underlying process of developing RSD. If we can understand this process, then options to cure RSD may come about more rapidly. Dr. Schwartzman and medical professionals working with him appear to be well on their way, and there is real hope among patients for what is to come.

Early detection, correct diagnosis and proper treatment within the first six to nine months override all other issues. If caught and treated properly early on, your chance of long-term remission is greatly increased according to many health sources. Therefore, prompt and proper treatments are the best way to control the severity and progression of RSD. The earlier we catch RSD, the better the chances for that patient to have a good outlook in controlling the RSD or putting it into remission. As the RSD in you progresses and is not addressed or is incorrectly treated, the issues become more complex and invasive. Patients who have had little response to fewer invasive procedures such as physical therapy have a greater chance that their symptoms will persist. It is most probable that the emotional factor plays a greater role and requires additional treatment in this area.

RSD patients find the best overall treatment with a team of professionals to manage all of the aspects of the syndrome. In my case, I have a pain specialist, neurologist, physical therapist (PT), pharmacist and a primary care physician (PCP) who are in contact with each other. Only one doctor should be dispensing your medications in this situation. I have chosen my primary care doctor. He receives all of the reports from the other team members and it is easiest for him to help me decide on what medications are working. Also, he and my pharmacist help detect any problems with drug interactions. Prior to having one doctor take control of my medications, I had many complications that resulted in hospital stays. Therefore, both doctor and patient should be involved in setting goals for the treatment and medications taken.

It is important to learn about the types of treatments available to you. Treatment options include physical therapy, medication, orthopedic surgery, invasive surgery and non-invasive procedures. Patients should look for ways to control and minimize pain and discomfort to the greatest extent possible. Coping skills will develop out of necessity with chronic pain patients. However, we sometimes need to speak to someone on the outside for a different view. Psychological counseling may become necessary. It is okay to ask for help. Goal creation and treatment plans should also include: drug management, family/social adjustment, improvement of the patient's quality of life and psychosocial functioning, and increasing mobilization or range of motion through physical therapy to help prevent progression and aggravation of RSD symptoms. It is important to treat the underlying symptoms even if it means turning to surgical intervention as a last possible option. Depending on how well you respond to the various options, a progression of treatments will be determined. In general, the initial treatments include nerve blocks, medication trials, medical team coordination, and physical therapy.

Pain specialists may become involved at the beginning of treatment or sometime after your PCP recommends. The pain doctor may be able to offer complementary therapies that may also be initiated at any point. Physical therapy and medications are commonly used as harmonizing therapies in the beginning of treatments. If there is no relief from the physical therapy within one to two months, then sympathetic nerve blocks (SNBs) may be considered. The SNBs are done in conjunction with drug therapy. The drug therapy may include nerve medications and lighter pain medications. This may offer enough pain relief to begin physical therapy exercises you could not do before. If no lasting relief after six weeks is achieved, a stronger, longer lasting narcotic, like morphine for breakthrough pain, along with anti-depressants, is usually prescribed. The anti-depressants are used for pain control as well as to treat the psychological effects related to prolonged pain and loss of enjoyment of life. Another way to treat RSD is through Ketamine or Lidocaine infusions that are effective for approximately 85% of in-patient patients.[7] A few patients also get an Intrathecal pump with bupivacaine and clonidine supplementation, and Intrathecal pump of Baclofen is often successful for severe Dystonia.

---

[7] Sandra P. Kofflera , Benjamin M. Hampstead, c, Farzin Iranid, Jennifer Tinkerd, Ralph-Thomas Kiefere, Peter Rohrf and Robert J. Schwartzman, The Neurocognitive Effects Of 5 Day Anesthetic Ketamine For The Treatment Of Refractory Complex Regional Pain Syndrome National Academy of Neuropsychology Published by Elsevier Ltd., Accepted 22 May 2007, information updated Oct, 2008

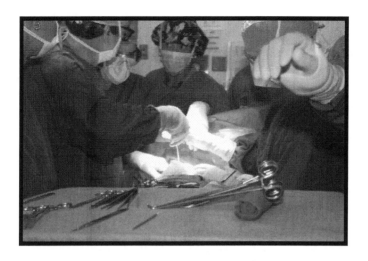

If there is any severe pain, working out is not recommended. In the case of RSD, pain is NO GAIN. Physical therapy should not be excruciating; know your limits, and do not be afraid to speak up. In my situation, not speaking up caused me more pain and worsened my symptoms. Don't let this happen to you. Physical therapy for RSD patients who are still in severe pain should include traction, stretching and massage, no weights. Therapy should be done to alleviate or lower pain levels, restore function to the limb, reduce swelling, reduce stiff joints, and strengthen muscles. If you do not use your limb, you will lose it. I know it can be very difficult to find the balance of physical therapy that helps you versus what hurts you. Make sure to find a PT who specializes in chronic pain and in RSD specifically, if possible. If the exercise does not feel right, speak up and do not do it. Have open communication with your physical therapist so you get the greatest benefits. You don't want to lose your limb, even though some days you may not want it attached to you either.

Accomplishing the goals of physical therapy begins with patient awareness. You need to use the limb despite the pain for as much as you can handle without having to pay for it in the following hours and days. Setting goals and a timetable that is reasonable can be done with your therapist. On your good days, try a few new things in your environment and increase your amount of physical activity. This can increase function, range of motion, and muscle strength and improve balance and posture. For me, as the pain gets worse, I find myself slouching more. Becoming aware of yourself and your environment greatly increases your chances of successful treatment of RSD and a better quality of life. Get involved in movement training. This can include walking for two minutes at a time or, if you're really ambitious, a mile. Do what you can do at your level. It will be different for all of us. Moving will increase your health and the function of your affected limbs, and it also helps with constipation and gastrointestinal issues caused by the RSD and medications. Movement increases your blood circulation, which helps with atrophy and can decrease hypersensitivity.

Using a combined therapy approach can give you faster relief. When most people think of physical therapy they think of machines and weights. However, I learned that there are many types of therapy that fall under the same realm of "physical". These therapies are more in line with what we are able to handle. The other physical therapy methods include biofeedback, hot compresses, elevation, massage, range of motion exercises, and hydrotherapies. There is some thought that physical therapy is painful and does not help. Patients can combine counseling, physical therapy and a drug regimen for better relief. Doing this can help us stay on track with our treatment plan and increase the benefits of physical therapy. Again, it comes back to surrounding yourself with a team of doctors, caretakers, and family supporters that have the education on RSD to support you.

One of the hardest things of this syndrome is the inability to work. Until it was gone from my life, I did not realize how important work was. Work provides a financial stability but also helps our sense of purpose. Having a purpose, or a sense of being needed, gave me a self-esteem boost and a better quality of life. One of the biggest things that helped me emotionally after RSD was finding things that I could do to help others. Although I received my degree in Social Psychology from George Mason University, my life was focused and prepared around cheerleading, dance and gymnastics. I did not train for anything else; I had no fall back plan. It was hard for me to go from working nonstop to being inactive. That is what RSD can do to you. I lost a lot of friends, and my social life became nonexistent. One therapy to think about when you are in this situation is occupational therapy. This is an important step in gaining back and seeing new ways to be an active and productive member of society. With RSD, you have to become creative in your everyday life situations. If you need someone to cut your food so it is easier to eat, you could return the favor by first thanking them and then offering to do something that you are able to do, like tutor their child in math or read them a book.

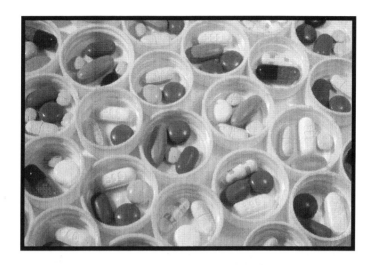

Medications will become a large part of your life as they are used to enhance effectiveness of treatments and to lower pain levels. It is important to be on a schedule with your medications as pain can intensify and side effects from the medications can occur. Keeping a steady level of the medication in your body instead of letting it go up and down from missed or late use will help keep your pain level under greater control. There are many drugs available to help us with pain. Remember, not all medications are right for you. I have been prescribed over twenty-five different medicines in one year alone while trying to find what works best for me.

Some pain relieving medications are:

- Anticonvulsants: Carbamazepine (Tegretol), Gabapentin (Neurontin), Phenytoin (Dilantin)
- Antidepressants: amitriptyline, Nortriptyiline
- Aspirin and Acetaminophen (Tylenol)
- Corticosteroids: to reduce inflammation and swelling, for example- Calcitonin spray
- Intrathecal Drug Delivery- Drugs delivered into the spinal fluid through the spinal cord or delivered through a pain pump- Pain pump drugs include morphine and Baclofen.[8]
- Muscle Relaxants: Baclofen (Lioresal), Klonopin
- Narcotic analgesics - usually reserved for severe, chronic pain
- Non-steroidal anti-inflammatory drugs (NSAIDs) or Ibubrophen
- Oral Opioids: used with widespread pain

My treatment plan from 2005 to 2009 is having a Radiofrequency (RF) procedure on a 5-6 week basis, and I

---

[8] It is important to note the implantation of a morphine pump is also associated with potential complications including: infection, bleeding, spinal fluid leaks, malfunction of the pump and injury to the spinal cord.

receive a sympathetic nerve block (SNB) along with my RF treatment through which I get relief. Although not all of my symptoms or pain goes away, the relief is priceless. Other people experience pain relief from just a SNB depending upon the severity of the RSD. The SNB does not block motor activity so you can remain mobile and active which offers you better range of motion. Your range of motion and exercises can increase during the time the nerve block has reduced the degree of pain.

My doctor also cautions me every time about the risks in undergoing the RF. Risks include new nerve injuries, bleeding, allergic reactions to the medications being used, seizures, and the stress and fear about the procedure. It is important that you have a competent pain management specialist because of the variety of complications involved in performing the procedure. My pain specialist happens to be an anesthesiologist who is experienced with the RF technique and is comfortable performing it on me. I suggest that you only get a RF procedure from a trained professional who treats RSD patients specifically and has performed this procedure on a regular basis. I have other symptoms after my procedure that my doctor reports are not common. It is important to notify your doctor of any side effects you may have or complications noted after the procedure. Further complications may develop or become life threatening if not taken care of when they first begin. After the procedure, I have a low-grade fever, stiff neck, general achiness for up to seven days, and basic flu like symptoms before the pain decreases.

Some doctors will try to go from a successful SNB or RF to a chemical or surgical Sympathectomy. A Sympathetomy involves cutting out the sympathetic ganglion nerve bundle, which is located in a specific area along the spinal cord. Once the nerve bundle is removed, there is nothing for the doctor to treat if the pain returns. Sympathectomy is a procedure that has high risks, and the outcome varies from patient to patient; this should be used as a last resort. Carefully weigh the risks of the procedure and communicate with your doctor in great detail. If it is determined that the source of the RSD pain is sympathetically maintained, in which pain is reduced with a sympathetic nerve block (SNB), then this may be an option. However, if the pain is determined to be sympathetically independent pain, a Sympathectomy is not a procedure that will benefit you. Once performed, the removal is permanent. Even if you have SMP, it may turn into SIP down the road with the additional trauma to the body, so the risks of failure are high for this procedure. If you have chosen to receive a full Sympathectomy, you will be limited or out of treatment options. With the possible risks, make sure that you are an appropriate candidate for this procedure and that you are willing to undergo the procedure in spite of the risks. Remember, this procedure does not always work even when the RSD is sympathetically driven.

There are multiple types of Sympathectomy procedures, including surgical and chemical. A surgical sympathetomy involves surgically cutting the nerves of the sympathetic ganglion at a specific location along the spinal cord. Your desired outcome is to suppress or block the SMP in the affected area. The chemical version uses a chemical that destroys the sympathetic ganglion nerve bundle. The most commonly used chemicals for this procedure are Phenol and Ethanol. Side effects from this include inflammation of the nerve and paralysis.

The procedure that I received every six weeks, radio-frequency ablation, is technically considered a Sympathectomy. The radiofrequency (RF) ablation uses radio-frequency heat to collapse veins around nerve tissue, which decreases pain signals and allows me to experience partial relief. My high pain levels return after four to six weeks as the nerves reawaken. Patients may have complete relief or no relief at all. Although most patients do experience complete or partial relief for several months, the effects are not lasting. The burning pain during this time is reduced for me after those few days of flu-like symptoms. Only a small percent (15-30%) experience long-term relief lasting two years or longer. In a study published in 2002 in the Journal of Vascular Surgery, researchers from the University Of South Florida College Of Medicine reported that patients had at least 50% reduction in pain intensity after a Sympathectomy. Only a small percent of patients reported no relief at all and are considered treatment failures.[9]

The post Radiofrequency pain I experience is associated with the surgical aspects of the procedure, which has been reported to occur in about 40% of patients. Other symptoms I notice after my procedure are excessive sweating, increase in my Horner's syndrome and extremely

---

[9] Journal of Vascular Surgery, researchers from the University of South Florida College of Medicine

low blood pressure after the procedure is finished. Horner's syndrome is a syndrome caused by injury to the sympathetic nerves of the face, which includes a constricted pupil, drooping eyelids, and facial dryness. Below is a picture of me when my Horner's Syndrome was very apparent.

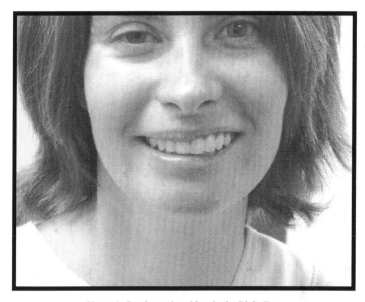

Horner's Syndrome is evident in the Right Eye

Other patients have also reported post Radiofrequency symptoms like pneumothorax, seizures and a recurrence or worsening of the RSD pain. Be sure to find a surgeon with experience and a high success rate with any of the Sympathectomy procedures before you schedule one for yourself.

An additional option is the use of a tens unit, which is also known as a nerve stimulator. The tens unit provides electrical nerve stimulation that, in small amounts to the nerves, overcomes the sensation of pain. It is a trick to your nerves. Think about when you have hurt yourself on something in the past. Your reaction is to rub the area. This causes a good sensation to be sent to the brain, which can sometimes help forget the pain. This does not always work, but the tens unit has been beneficial to me. I use the tens unit because it is non-invasive. Mine is battery-operated, portable and available for self-treatment because it is a small unit. I can use it as needed and can place the electrodes where I need them most. Although I have not experienced negative effects from the tens unit, some people get skin rashes from the sticky side of the electrode. Also, people with pacemakers and pregnant women should not use the tens unit or the spinal cord stimulator.

There is another option to surgically place a spinal cord stimulator with lead wires into the epidural space in your spinal column attached to an external controller. You can also use a Peripheral nerve stimulator for similar use. What is different about a Peripheral nerve stimulator from the spinal cord stimulator is that the electrodes are placed outside the central nervous system and target the peripheral nervous system. For both types of stimulators, small wires are implanted and can move; however they can be placed in a position where they may not be helpful. There are many other complications such as infections and the higher risk of spreading of RSD to other parts of your body.

Spinal cord stimulators (SCS) have an effect on the entire central nervous system. The idea with this choice is having the spinal cord interrupt the pain signal to the brain. Before a SCS is implanted permanently, you should have a period with a temporary stimulator. This trial period should last for several days to a week. If you have a positive result from the temporary stimulator, your doctor may ask if you want to go to the next step of permanent implantation. The surgical implantation is described as feeling like an electrical current but is reported by patients to be far less bothersome compared to the pain of RSD. When one of my doctors suggested this as a future option, I tried to remain open-minded. Just the thought of it scared me enough. I considered it by looking at the reported risks and complications. This helped me make my mind up really quickly. The spinal stimulator is not a cure, but in many cases, it can reduce the pain to a more manageable level. However, only a small number of RSD patients who have the stimulator have benefits that last more than 2 years, and most patients have complications such as moved leads, infections, quick drainage of power from batteries, and feeling of internal shocks in your spine. Any patients that are undergoing radiation, have pacemakers or are exposed to alarm detection devices should not consider this option. Alarm detection devices include security sites at airports, aircraft communications systems and anti-theft devices in stores.

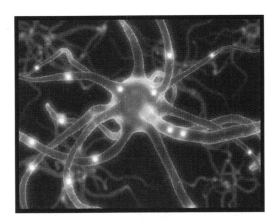

Healthy Communication on neurological level

Complications associated with surgical implantation of the SCS include:

- Significant bleeding in the epidural space
- Infection in the epidural space that can lead to meningitis or an epidural abscess. This may require a surgical procedure to treat the problem. Any infection in the epidural space would require removal of the spinal cord stimulator system.
- Tenderness at the Generator/Receiver which is common until healing occurs, but persistent pain at the stimulator site is possible, as is tissue damage at the site of the SCS lead and connecting cable(s)
- Surgical complications associated with SCS, which includes injury to the spinal cord, paralysis, accumulation of fluid in the power source site (Seroma), and spinal headaches
- Mechanical complications with the system, including dislodgement or movement of the lead, breaks in the wiring or with the power source
- Occasionally, loss of pain relief in a painful area, even if stimulation is still felt in that area[10]

---

[10] Seacoastpain.com, Spinal Cord Stimulation Informed Consent Information, SPI 2006

Other treatment options for RSD patients include topical pain patches; I used Lidoderm patches as well as Lidocaine lotion. Other topical medications used are Fontanel and Clonidine. Be sure to check with your doctor about potential side effects. Some RSD patients also use acupuncture as a treatment. I am weary of this because any trauma to the body can increase your symptoms and cause additional problems. Other adverse issues with acupuncture include: bleeding, inflammation, intensification of pain, nerve irritation and or injury, infections, poor wound healing, and skin irritations.

The good news is that no matter how long you have had RSD you can be helped in some way, as long as you are willing to stay active, are able to avoid surgical procedures, can change medication usage when needed and will improve eating habits. Unfortunately, RSD affects many systems of the body over time, the autonomic and central nervous system, immune system, limbic, gastrointestinal and more. Patients can convince themselves that a doctor or surgeon has the ability to perform surgery on them that will cure them. In the beginning, I was one of these patients myself.

Resorting to surgery can lead an RSD patient to a wheelchair and the need for larger doses of narcotic medication at an accelerated rate. As of now, there is no quick fix for RSD. There is not even a great treatment method that works for all patients. In 1983, Dr. Poplawski from Canada published a study about the outcome of RSD. He showed that RSD diagnosed in the first two years has a chance of successful treatment in 80% of the patients, and after two years, each year drops the percentage of the success significantly.[11] Other doctors say within the first six to nine months is the window for remission.

---

[11] Poplawski ZJ, Wiley AM, Murray JF: Post traumatic dystrophy of the extremities. J Bone Joint Surg [Am] 1983; 65:642-55

Many RSD patients consider these milestones as successful
treatment of RSD:

- Ability to achieve a full night's sleep repeatedly
- Ability to perform physical therapy with marked improvement in muscle strength
- Decreased need for narcotics
- Diminished depression
- Diminished swelling of the effected arm or leg
- Improved thinking
- Increased stamina
- Lowered pain levels, or pain controlled with low to moderate consideration

EMOTIONAL ASPECTS OF RSD

Mental health can be disrupted with RSD. Anxiety, depression, feeling of hopelessness, isolation and helplessness can increase to dangerous levels. Particularly for people who have been suffering with RSD for a long period of time, life can become overwhelming. When I finally realized that RSD had no cure and that my future would include pain on a daily basis, I began to have dark thoughts. I do not want to end up at the risk of suicide. There are going to be good and bad days, and if this is a bad day for you, remember to focus on the good days, good feelings and positive past and future experiences. It is very important for you and your family to recognize the symptoms of diminished emotional well-being and take action.

Understand that these feelings and thoughts are common among RSD'ers. It is helpful to create an overall strategy to get through the rough times. RSD patients learn over time that they can better cope and adjust to both the physical and psychological consequences of the disorder with the help and support of spiritual guidance, family and

83

therapists. Creating an arsenal of tools, such as spirituality, physical modalities and meditation, are all ways to better your situation. Turning to God has especially helped me with anxiety, depression and other psychological and physical challenges, and it offers a great way to cope with and put situations into proper perspective so we can learn to live with it.

RSD is not understood very well, and there are physicians and psychiatrists who believe that it is all in our heads or that people just complain for the sake of workmen's compensation issues. If we are seen as malingering patients who just won't go away, doctors who don't understand RSD may find it difficult to look for any other diagnosis other than psychological. A lot of my stress could have been avoided if doctors had really listened to me from the start instead of looking at my marriage troubles as an excuse to "be ill for attention."

With the loss of independence and function, it is hard for many patients to accept their changing life. Be sure to surround yourself with a team who is on your side, or you will be in a fight in which you will have trouble winning. I went through a grieving process in the course of coming to grips with my new reality. This is not uncommon for RSD patients.

There were stages to my grieving. First was hope. I hoped that there was some cure to make the pain go away. Second, wondering if the treatment I was receiving was appropriate, I got angry. The feeling of resentment and depression from when I realized that this is not temporary is sometimes overwhelming in itself. When this happens, I try to rationalize and evaluate the changes in my life and how I live it. In doing this I come to an understanding and acceptance of what my place is with the permanent pain.

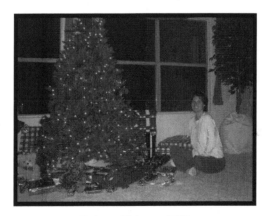

Barby on Christmas, 2005

It is important that patients with RSD and other chronic pain conditions maintain a healthy lifestyle, including getting enough sleep, exercising, and eating healthy foods, despite the difficulties we experience. There are long-term health consequences created by our changing lifestyle because of RSD. As patients with RSD, we typically lead a more sedentary lifestyle due to our pain. Because we are less active, we are at greater risk for developing other medical problems. I myself have been dealing with poor posture and sudden weight gain and loss. I fall easily and have trouble gripping and holding onto things. In the long term we need to watch out for cardiovascular disease, diabetes and osteoporosis as the risk for these conditions is heightened with inactivity.

Weight control is my biggest issue. As a former athlete, I know it is crucial for good health. Nutrition also plays a role in RSD and how we prepare our bodies to cope with the stress on us every day. Make sure that your doctor is doing frequent blood testing to check for any deficiencies you may develop. Medications can also affect your liver, kidneys and digestive system. Blood testing can help prevent this from getting out of control as well as let you know if there are any vitamin supplements you may need to take to counter poor absorption. Try finding clubs and workout facilities that offer programs for physically handicapped individuals, or use things around your house if you do not get out often, as is the case for me.

I try to use my affected arm as much as possible. I tend to shield my arm from any stimulation and from being touched or manipulated due to the increase in pain levels, even from the smallest of stimuli. This is something to overcome and find solutions around. For instance, my caretakers assist me in bathing and other activities that are painfully overwhelming for me. Maintaining good hygiene may be painful but is very important. My new reality is that I am disabled and do need to ask for help. This is also part of a cycle. Every new doctor, therapist and even talk of a new treatment from other patients gives me that hope once again. I now understand that healing is a process, and I have control with how I look at life my life. The cycle of grief is shown through anger, resentment, depression, understanding, hope and then acceptance.

I have found that patients with RSD, including myself, experience depression, fear, anxiety and anger. The idea of living with this horrible syndrome with no cure is astounding. A study by the International Association for the Study of Pain recommends that psychological intervention be initiated for patients experiencing pain for more than two months.[12] When my experience with RSD started, I was already in therapy for personal reasons, but it soon became apparent that my nameless symptoms were taking over my life, and I was unable to focus on anything but coping with "the new me." When doctors told me, "Just do this and you will be okay," I would build up my hope and follow their directions. When I did not get better, I came crashing down, and so did life around me. I have since gone to therapy on and off throughout my process of learning to live with RSD. I tried group therapy and found it to be better than one-on-one counseling for me. Hearing that I was not the only one out there in this large world gave me a peace.

Relaxation and meditation techniques I had learned in my sessions help me reduce muscle spasms, pain, and improve my dysfunctional sleeping patterns. Learning to LIVE with pain and still accomplish life goals is an important part of treatment. Counseling helps me cope, raises my self-esteem and prepares me mentally to take on RSD instead of allowing RSD to take me. Having positive

---

[12] Physical Medicine and Rehabilitation Review, Pg 179, International Association for the Study of Pain, Contributor Robert J. Kaplan, Published by McGraw-Hill, 2005

thoughts, even self-given, helps me remain positive and change my behavior and emotional state.

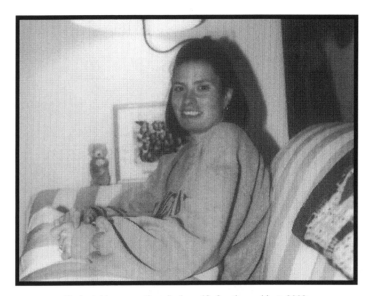

Barby taking some time for herself after the accident, 2002

This biofeedback is a way to train our bodies to improve our health. We can use signals both visually and auditory from our own bodies to improve our condition. This is a powerful tool that gives us some choice in our reaction to our pain. Biofeedback can also help with blood pressure, heart rate, muscle tension and body temperature, which all contribute to our chronic pain. Many doctors report better outcomes with patients who use this biofeedback technique. Lowering anxiety and fear and the ability to relax through the tough times help us cope better with the chronic pain. Practicing coping techniques like meditation, deep breathing, visual imaging, yoga and other such relaxing activities on a daily basis will help us improve our pain control. This improvement will allow us to be in command of our own life as well as reduce our pain levels. Calming the mind and body through mental relaxation will improve our function; we just have to do it consistently and effectively. I have found that keeping a positive attitude helps me cope with the pain as well as the daily stresses in life. Adopting positive thinking as a way of life can help lower the pain levels as well as help you with stress and anxiety-filled situations. When I am in a stressful situation or face a life challenge, I find it brings constructive changes if I look at the situation in an optimistic light. Optimism is confidence, hopefulness and a cheerful way of coping with a challenge that is seemingly daunting. To me, optimism is believing that things are continually getting better and that good will ultimately prevail over evil.

Creating a positive attitude starts with being inspired. Begin by finding an interest or hobby you can become involved with and will enjoy. A few suggestions are joining a non-profit cause, solving puzzles, writing a journal, joining or starting a support group, or even starting a blog. Creating a purpose can assist with your self-esteem and confidence. Just because you are disabled does not mean you are not worth anything. I have learned that every person has a value no matter how big or small. Believing in yourself and in your abilities, choosing happiness and thinking creatively is good motivation when it comes to accomplishing your goals. Expect success when you are going through your daily activities. It might take you longer or you may need to use more constructive thinking to achieve success, but it is possible.

Negative situations are bound to appear, but when you are looking for solutions and displaying self-esteem and confidence, you will also attract other people to participate in helping you accomplish your needs and goals. Try looking at failure and problems as blessings in disguise. Doing so will help solutions find you. Seize the opportunities in everyday life. Using your outings to inform others of your condition, finding pleasure in your minor accomplishments, and not giving up are just a few ways to increase your power of positive thinking.

There are great benefits to having a positive attitude. Especially when things are not going your way, staying optimistic will allow you more energy, happiness and lower pain levels. Achieving goals is a great motivator for positive thinking. Success is achieved faster and more easily through positive thinking, and it will inspire and motivate you and others. I have found that when I am letting the pain get the better of me, it comes across to others as disrespect and brings those around me down.

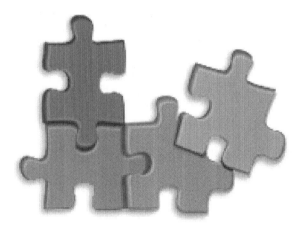

Staying calm and positive creates an atmosphere for greater inner strength and power. You can also create better communication with a calm positive attitude, which will assist you in working with your doctors and caretakers. When you take life one task at a time and approach each challenge with optimism, it leads to fewer difficulties encountered along the way and increases the ability to overcome any difficulty. As my father always says when I am having a bad day, "Tomorrow will be a better day."

No matter the challenges of today, they will pass, and in retrospect, they will not seem as bad as time moves on. The challenges may just turn out to be a bump that looked like a mountain at the time. Remez Sasson says, "Positive attitude helps us to cope more easily with the daily affairs of life. It brings optimism into your life, and makes it easier to avoid worry and negative thinking. If you adopt it as a way of life, it will bring constructive changes into your life, and makes them happier, brighter and more successful."[13] I have found that when I live life with a negative attitude I am saying that I do not respect myself and do not believe success is possible. Try working on displaying a positive attitude and the moods of others and

---

[13] The Power of Positive Attitude, Remez Sasson, successconsciousness.com

the challenges of life will become easier to deal with. Choosing to be happy starts with you. No person or thing can make you happy and positive. It is a skill you have to practice and develop when living with chronic pain. When you are able to live in a happy, positive and optimistic light, your life will become a life worth the ups and downs that come with it.

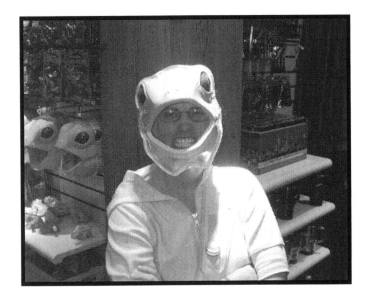

RECAP

- Choose happiness.
- Create goals and more towards accomplishing them.
- Get involved in projects that you can be interested in and successfully complete.
- Keep yourself surrounded with happy people.
- Look at the bright side of challenges.
- Motivate yourself.
- Practice meditation and controlling your thoughts.
- Smile big and often.
- Visualize success.
- When anxiety and stresses are high, turn it over to God.

ROLES PEOPLE IN YOUR LIFE WILL PLAY

Creating a support system in your life is a must! Your support system can take the form of your family, friends, a support group, healthcare providers, and caretakers. You may find it beneficial to map out a plan of action with your support team so that a daily routine is established and maintained. This can serve to minimize stress levels when unexpected changes in plans arise.

When you have chronic pain, making life as stress free as possible is important. Of course, you are changing inside. As you change physically and mentally, the people around you must also adjust. As they do, you may find that they do not fit into your life the same way or at all. Some people cannot handle watching someone else in pain and feel bad that they cannot fix it. They may tend to react by cutting you off or ignoring you. They may also compensate by bullying you or babying you. The reality of your new situation is that as the change is taking place on the inside, you must also deal with the outside. You can make positive changes with dealing and communicating with others in your life and the new roles assumed by you and them.

Transforming our world so that our most precious resources on the inside work together with our outer influences will help us with our new daily reality. Changing your approach to situations and your perspective makes you see things from a different angle. You can prepare and react to the new roles that those around you take on. Learning to use the people in your life to better your situation will also help them stay positive, and they can play larger roles in your life, whether it means backing off from some people or embracing offers from others. Limiting your time, discussions or interactions with particular people in your life will help everyone cope with stress of your new disability.

Look at your life as different, not over. Try arousing your hidden inner potential by trying new activities, learning new subjects and working to create balance and harmony between how you feel and what you can do. Bring out the good qualities that you have hidden inside you by experiencing the freedom of being your genuine self. When you're in pain it is hard to be anything but your true self; it can expose the raw side of who you are. The pain has helped me gain self-knowledge, avoid unnecessary detours in life and cultivate love and goodness in myself and in those I choose to have around me. By my learning to manage pain, fear and anger, I have been able to create new circumstances and enjoy a better life quality, allowing those around me to also become better people. Paying attention to how you are living and reacting has many positive advantages. It has helped me become the person I want to be towards others in my life as well as become more spiritual. It has been helpful in refining my values. Living in pain has given me the chance to experience real satisfaction and happiness, forgive myself, and love and embrace myself on a grand level.

How can you take the step in using those in your life to assist you, without taking advantage of them? Start with making a list of what needs to be done. Decide what you can do on the list and what you need assistance with. Responsibilities that need to be considered include: cleaning, cooking, laundry, mail drop off and delivery, pet care, planning meals, shopping, social activities and transportation. Below are tips to accomplish tasks of daily living.

- Cleaning
  - Ask others to assist with the heavy work such as vacuuming and mopping.
  - Choose one room every few days to concentrate on picking up or dusting.
  - Hire a cleaning service.
  - Put items away as you use them.
- Transportation
  - Bring extra medication with you in case you have a flare up.
  - Double check times, dates and locations of appointments before you leave the house.
  - Use pillows and blankets to stay warm and comfortable.
- Shopping
  - Have a plan as to what you are looking for and what you want to accomplish while you are out.
  - Use assistive devices that allow you to use less energy so you're able to shop longer.

- Cooking
  - Have someone cut food for you (or buy precut food) and store in small containers for easy use when needed.
  - Make small meals.
  - Split up larger items into small, more manageable containers.
- Laundry
  - Have someone assist with folding, ironing and putting away the clothes.
  - Sort laundry as it is dirtied (whites, colors, to be dry-cleaned).
  - Wash more frequently.
  - Wash smaller loads.
- Planning Meals
  - Choose items easy to make.
  - Choose items that have a longer shelf life.
  - Keep items on lower shelves.
  - Order items from stores with home delivery.

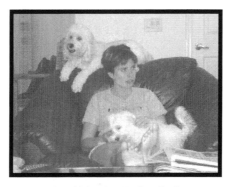

Barby with her dog, Tuci, on her lap;
She was unable to take care of him and adopted him out to a family in 2004

- Pet Care
  - Ask neighborhood kids to take the dog for a walk or play with him in the park.
  - Install a doggie door.
  - Use larger food bowls so that they do not need to be filled as often.
- Mail Drop off and Delivery
  - Prepare your bills and outgoing mail so that next time you go out or someone comes to visit, it is ready to go and easily dealt with.
  - The delivery guy can carry the items into your house instead of dropping them on the porch.

- Social Activities
  - Choose creative activities you enjoy and are less physically demanding.
  - Let the people attending know that you have good and bad days or moments and you may not be able to make it, may leave early or come late.
  - Let them know ahead of time if you need quiet space.
  - Let them know how you want to be greeted such as a hug, air hug, hand shake, or head nod.

CHANGE IN FAMILY DYNAMICS

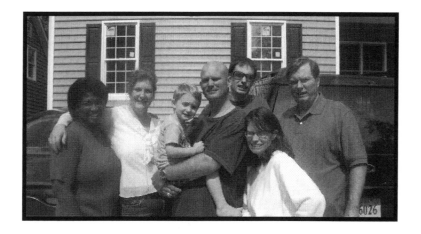

Reflex Sympathetic Dystrophy (RSD) can be a lifelong condition that has a significant impact not only on the patient but on family and friends as well. The condition may affect many aspects of the patient's life in varying degrees including activities of daily living, professional, social and personal life. The patient will have to make some adjustments. After health, patients are usually hit hardest in the financial aspects of this chronic disorder. They frequently need a leave of absence from work or possibly early retirement due to inability or difficulty performing work-related tasks. With less money and mobility they tend to give up or modify leisure activities such as hiking, kayaking, traveling, and participating in family activities and outings. Exercising becomes difficult, if not impossible, to manage. Everyday activities such as driving and shopping have to be given up or modified. Financial difficulties are acerbated due to frequent visits to health-care providers, medical-related expenses and unemployment.

Friends and family may find it beneficial to map out a plan of action with the patient's participation so that a daily routine is established. This reduces stress levels and minimizes unexpected changes in plans. Responsibilities that may need to be addressed include:

- Car pools
- Chores/housework
- Cooking
- Holiday activities
- Jobs (employment)
- Laundry
- Leisure activities

- Pet care
- Planning meals
- Self care
- Sex life
- Shopping
- Social life

The patient should be encouraged to stay active and to join a support group or seek psychological counseling if appropriate. Patients may even reach the point of ultimately counseling others with RSD. Some patients find benefit in getting involved in volunteer work, which allows them to set their own hours and to feel that they still can contribute to others instead of just focusing on their own condition.

Despite a wide range of treatment options available to patients with RSD, some patients do not seek help since they may be discouraged by constant pain and are worn down both physically and emotionally. This may result in their dismissing efforts by others to help them. Some of their concerns include:

- Fear of side effects from treatments
- Fear that nothing can help them

- Fear that they will be seen as "complainers" if they talk about their pain
- Fear that they will become addicted to medications
- Fear that they will develop a tolerance to medications and the recurring pain will be even worse

It is important to discuss these concerns with family members, friends, physicians, or support service professionals (e.g., psychologist, social worker), in order to take advantage of options that are available and may actually lead to pain relief and improvement in the overall quality of life. I can see how it is difficult (or impossible) to imagine that someone can be in severe pain continually if one has not experienced it. It is normal for you not to understand it if you have not lived through it. I did not understand and as a former athlete, it was hard to talk about pain and what I was going through. Society also does not often address the issues around chronic pain either. I often hear "you look healthy," but often I suffer excruciating, unforgiving, and burning pain.

For a caretaker, it may be hard to stand by and accept that your loved one's pain cannot be fixed or cured (although it may be eased). It may also be hard to accept that you cannot make it better. If you are in a close relationship with someone with chronic pain, you are likely to develop a variety of negative feelings as a result. This is a normal part of the process. Your emotions can range from anger to resentment. Both you and the loved one in pain are victims of the pain problem. Significant lifestyle changes will affect the caretaker; for instance: time, social support, outside intrusions, and reduced income.

- Anxiety and guilt due to financial problems that result from your loved one's disability and the realization you can't help cure them
- As a result of a withdrawal of affection or a decline in your sex life, you may develop depression.
- You get angry if the person is irritable or withdrawn.
- You may become resentful having to take over tasks they previously performed.
- You take on stress because of others' reactions. For example, "he doesn't look that disabled to me" or "why doesn't he want to work?"

Family and friends often become caretakers for the patient in pain and are also victims of the pain problem. Both patients and caretakers experience reduced social support and intrusions into your life. For example, some insurance companies may follow or film you and your families, thinking that you are all in on faking for financial gain. Your family may have a reduction of income or have to work harder to stay afloat financially to make up for the lost wages of the patient. Due to reduced income, unemployment, and medical expenses required for various treatments, family income can be cut in half or diminish to nothing. It may be shrewd for the patient and their family to meet with a financial planner or an insurance agent and devise a budget so that future and unexpected expenses will be accounted for. This may reduce the general stress level for the patient and their loved ones.

This can become a harsh reality. I lost my job and had no income of my own. My family and caretakers had to help me out or I would become indigent. Until my social security disability kicked in, I was basically at the mercy of food stamps and family support. It is not only financially hard on direct family; often times extended family is asked to step in and help. If they cannot see the injury or they do not believe the patient in pain, it becomes very difficult. I have undergone significant lifestyle changes. I used to be able to do things like eating out often, cooking, shopping, driving, and cleaning. These activities are now challenges, both financially and physically. Again, turning to family and friends as caretakers and support outlets is important for the patient.

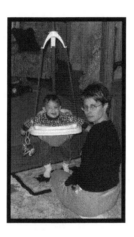

Remember, caretakers are also going through life changes because of supporting the patient. They now have to take time getting you to medical or other appointments if you cannot drive. They may end up doing most or all household chores and child-rearing activities. Understanding that this is hard on you and your caretakers is important for better communication. Caretakers may also experience some positive outcomes, although this is less common. If you were controlling, they may actually have to accept that they have more freedom, or if they have a very strong need to help others, they may feel good about helping you.

To have the caretakers take care of themselves first is most important. You cannot take care of someone else properly if you are not keeping yourself together. Try not to feel guilty when you need a break to do something for you. No one can be there for someone else around the clock. You can take care of yourself by choosing a healthy lifestyle that puts yourself first.

TIPS

- Discuss options with your loved one when he or she is ready to talk about them.
- Don't isolate yourself from friends and family.
- If prayer is helpful, keep doing it.
- If they are grouchy or depressed, don't see it as an attack on you but as a reflection of their pain.
- Keep exercising (or start).
- Learn as much as you can about the patient's

condition and the available medical options.

- Look for support wherever you can find it.
- Maintain a healthy lifestyle.
- Participate in religious or spiritual organization.
- Remember they are not doing this on purpose and are suffering just as you are.
- Socialize as much as possible.
- Join or make a support group for loved ones of patients with pain.
  - o This may be other family members or friends.
  - o This will allow you to take a break at times.
- Take in good nutrition.
- Try not to take your loved one's behavior personally.
- Try to avoid being either too babying or too harsh toward your loved one.
- Try to find others to help with the care of your loved one.
- Your loved one may also feel less guilty if the burden does not fall only on you!

When it comes to communication with the patient, try to avoid hurtful comments like, "you'll just have to live with it." Pay attention to your gestures and non-verbal communication. Rejection shows through actions as well as words. How you choose to say something, your tone of voice, facial expressions, and eye contact, or lack of, are all signs of rejection, resentment and show other negative feelings. When you see someone frowning or sneering, they do not have to say a word, and you can guess pretty well what is going through their mind. Your gestures communicate just as much as words do.

Communication with your family member in pain is a family challenge, not just an individual one. Try to see the disability as a challenge that you all face together. Take the approach of "we," not "he," will fight this together. Listening to what the patient is saying and watching what you say can keep the lines of communication open. Pretending to be interested when you are not can create a breakdown in communication and in your ability to help the other person and vice versa.

Be real with your emotions. If you do not believe, ask more questions, and get more information. It matters that you accept their pain to be as they say it is. Do not tell them "it can't be that bad" unless you are trying to hurt them and the situation. If you pay attention not only to what your loved one is saying, but to their nonverbal communication and how they are saying it, they may be less reluctant to talk about how they feel or give indications in their behavior as to how they are doing. If you have questions about your patient's pain reports, remember that chronic pain is rarely imaginary. You may question if they could be faking it to get out of work or some other challenge. Consciously faking pain to get out of something or to get a reward is known as malingering. While it does occur, it is rare. Most patients will feel very guilty about not being able to do the things they used to do, whether working at a job or doing chores around the house. Negative emotions from the patient or to the patient such as depressed mood, anger, or anxiety play an important role in increasing pain levels. When confronted with these emotions, be sure to recognize them but don't take them personally. For the patient, anxiety, stress and anger can cause an increase in muscle tension leading to more pain.

I am most helped in my chronic pain when those closest to me express concern for my suffering and offer help that is genuinely needed. Their encouragement for me to be as active as possible helps me stay social through rough days. As a caretaker, do not overdo your sympathy or try to remove all obstacles and challenges from someone in pain. On the other hand, do not punish the sufferer through blame and hostility. If you are not sure how best to be helpful, you might ask the person in pain what kind of attention they feel is most helpful and respectful. Judging how the patient is doing without asking them is going to be based on your perception and may not be accurate. Remember, people in pain learn coping skills as time goes on, and they may not be crying all the time but still have severe pain.

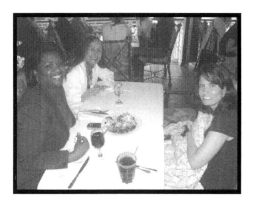

It is also helpful to me when people close to me show encouragement when I am trying to be as active as possible. I can tell when people are overdoing sympathy. I like to challenge myself but find that some people will try to remove all obstacles and challenges from me because I am in pain. On the other hand, I do not like being punished by blame and hostility when I am able to do something at a good moment and need help with the same task later. I like when people ask me what kind of attention and assistance I need. It feels helpful and respectful and puts me at ease.

My husband attends medical visits with me. When attending medical visits with me, he gets involved in the conversation when appropriate. Since meeting, before we even dated, he has only missed a handful of appointments. I have him ask the doctor what medications are prescribed, dosages, and how often I need to take them. I have had trouble in the past with overdosing or missing medication at times. With him knowing what the regimen is supposed to be, it helps me stay on track. When he understands what medication is prescribed and the overall treatment plan, he can better understand what I am going through. Also, RSD patients and pain patients in general, have trouble with short-term memory. This is caused by multiple factors. The sleep cycle is disturbed causing a lack of concentration. The medications they take make them groggy or less able to concentrate. For me, the biggest reason is that the pain is overwhelming. It is hard to concentrate when pain levels are high.

Having your caretaker taking notes at the doctor's office can remind them and the patient of important information about new medications, research to do, and approved activities. When I was in physical therapy, my husband asked questions and then worked with the PT on me to be able to perform traction and massage at home properly.

The healthcare provider and physical therapist can also help you understand what the appropriate level of activity is for your loved one. It is important to find the boundary between motivation and hurtful nudge. It is important to understand the overall treatment plan and help the pain patient stick to it. I have seen firsthand that dealing with severe pain can be overwhelming for both the patients and those who care for them. Working together with everyone involved will take some of the stress and anxiety off everyone. Try to be an advocate for your patient. Going to the doctor with a hidden agenda can make matters worse. For example, some people ask the doctor who prescribes the medications if he thinks they are necessary to undermine his authority. This type of attitude affects how the doctor sees the patient on a treatment level. Also, both the doctor and the patient can become isolated from you.

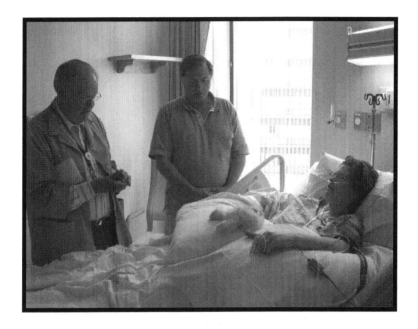

My mother worked in the healthcare industry until her recent retirement. She attended a doctor's appointment with me in Colorado and was with me during my first rib surgery in Arizona. She knows enough to try to help me, but in speaking up in the tone and manner with which she approached the doctors got to them. One even wrote a note in my records. The entire time I was in another surgery, my mother told my husband she had a bad feeling that things were done incorrectly by the doctors, all before I even got out of surgery. This scares the hell out of anyone. It is important to be positive about these situations once the decision is made to go forward. In the end, I did have complications on that surgery, but there is a better way to handle a stressful medical situation and a better way to approach the doctors. On the next surgery, I took my husband and my father, who also asked questions, but were there to support me in a positive manner. The doctor was much more receptive in sharing information and showed a genuine will to help. The problem is not asking questions; it is trying to meet your own agenda that breaks down patient and doctor communications. Advocating for your patient requires tact, unless of course they are in a dangerous situation.

One study evaluating quality of life issues among patients with RSD reported that the greatest interruption in daily life was related to activities of living.[14] The greatest disruptions in my daily life are directly related to pain, difficulty sleeping, and lack of energy. In the beginning, mobility was not a significant issue for me, but in 2006 I

---

[14] Health-Related Quality of Life in Chronic Refractory Reflex Sympathetic Dystrophy (Complex Regional Pain Syndrome Type I). Journal of Pain and Symptom Management, Volume 20, Issue 1, Pages 68 – 76, M. Kemler

began having RSD symptoms in my foot and began having problems with a greater range of symptoms. It increased the amount of coping needed to accomplish my daily activities.

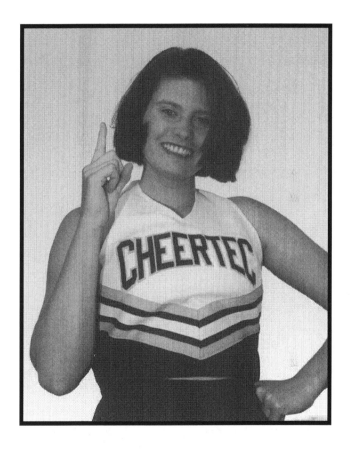

TIPS

Assessing how the patient is doing

- Are they able to communicate?
- Are they able to stay focused and remember things?
- Are they frequently grimacing, crying, groaning, or otherwise indicating extreme distress?
- Are they maintaining proper grooming practices?
- Are they sleeping at night for the right number of hours?
- Can they speak clearly and audibly and does what they say make sense?
- Do they appear anxious or irritable?
- Do they appear depressed?
- Has their appetite increased or decreased, or have they gained or lost weight?
- Have they increased use of tobacco or alcohol?
- Have they maintained their relationships with family and friends?
- Insomnia and poor sleeping cycles can result from being in a lot of pain.

Family and friends who form the support group around the patient must be educated and aware about RSD, its treatment and rehabilitation, behaviors of the patient that should be encouraged or discouraged, and supporting roles they can play. It is very important for friends and family to understand what the patient is going through and allow the patient the opportunity to express his or her grief and frustration without being judgmental. Family and friends also need to be supportive and to encourage the patient to keep his or her spirits up and to continue functioning to the best of his or her ability. Some patients become depressed if their condition prevents them from doing things that are important to their independence and well-being. Formerly independent people may have to rely on others for daily tasks (e.g., dressing, cooking, and errands). Having to have someone assist you is inconvenient and can make you feel you have a loss of self-respect. It is important to address these feelings and to respond appropriately.

WHAT DO YOU SAY

You can never take back information once it is shared but you can always wait to let people know later. If you choose to disclose that you have RSD, decide when and how to do so. If there is time to prepare ahead of time, it is a good idea. Take time to think about different situations and how you wish to handle them. Many people feel it is not their place to ask about your physical conditions, but knowing about RSD and chronic pain would help them understand where you are coming from with your thoughts and actions. When you are deciding to disclose your RSD and limitations, make the decision whether or not to let others know about your invisible disability. I know an RSD patient who liked a neighbor and was interested in dating him. He often helped around her house with handyman projects, and she would see him out on his porch and go out and talk to him. Eventually, he asked her out, and they had a great time. Over the next few months they had dates scheduled but she ended up canceling a lot of them. She was just in too much pain. He began to think she was not interested in him and started to pull away. Friends encouraged her to tell him about RSD and what she is going through. She did, and he stuck around for a while. In the end it did not work out, but they remained friends and it helped her see that you can still have a social life despite the RSD. If you're in this or another social situation you should think about the following when deciding to disclose your RSD and how it affects your everyday life. Are you able to participate in the activities at hand using your coping skills and tools? Do you need accommodations? Are you able to perform the activity safely if you choose not to disclose? Secondly, do you think they will react in a way appropriate for the environment you are in? If you are not sure, you may want to wait until you are in a private setting. If the situation becomes an intimate relationship, it is important to share even if it means losing the person. It is not fair to them or yourself to keep information back. If your disability is in remission or typically under control, is there a reason to disclose? Possibly the education you give them may help someone else they meet along the way. It is possible that flare-ups on your part may keep you from future activities. Finally, how will you address misconceptions about your disability when you disclose? Some people do not believe in treating pain with narcotic medications or have a bad experience with someone else in their life with chronic pain. Having them not understanding can lead to a divide. Also, not telling others is not an option if you are in a situation that can cause others harm. For instance, when getting on a plane, you cannot have the exit row. If assigned by mistake, notify the flight crew.

When choosing situations and activities where you do not want to disclose your disability, take time to carefully analyze the kind activities you are able to do and plan accordingly. Remember, you can always reveal more information later as needed. The following are some of the risks and benefits of letting others know about your disability.

RISKS

- Many RSD patients are seen as a drug or attention seeker, or as mentally unstable.
- You may face discrimination, subtle or direct, from work, friends and caretakers.
- You may face envy or resentment for receiving special treatment from the others in your life,

especially with children.

- You may not be asked to participate in the event or future activities, if the other person does not understand.

- You will have to give up your privacy to receive help bathing, eating and corresponding with others.

BENEFITS

- Letting others know about RSD can give you a sense of purpose and support for yourself and others in your life.

- Openness with your doctors, family and public can create understanding for others with invisible disabilities.

- You may be an ambassador for others with disabilities as a public educator, mentor or on a personal level.

- Your abilities, attitudes and success may counteract any discrimination. I think, if I keep doing what I can, they will eventually see. Even if they don't get it, you can still be successful.

Too many people misinterpret RSD. There are many physicians who are not familiar with the condition and its symptoms, and many who perceive their patients' complaints to be psychiatric in nature ("it's all in your head"). In addition, since RSD is related to many cases of workmen's compensation for injury occurring on the job or personal injury cases, there may be a tendency for some health care providers to view the patient's complaints as malingering. This is a significant source of stress for many patients, including myself, and may lead to significant delays in diagnosis and treatment. This situation adds to the psychosocial issues that we as patients already deal with due to chronic pain. It can disrupt quality of life and treatments.

As a patient, you may have to deal with a loss of independence as your level of functioning may be significantly compromised. It is hard for many patients to accept their changing condition. Many go through a grieving process in the course of coming to grips with their new reality.

Some medical literature describes seven stages through which people move in relating to chronic pain including:[15]

- Acceptance & hope
- Anger & bargaining
- Depression, reflection, loneliness
- Pain & guilt
- Reconstruction & working through
- Shock & denial
- The upward turn

As a pain patient, I have gone through the stages of grief with a slightly different perspective. I wondered if the treatment I was receiving was appropriate. I had, and still have, hope that there will someday be a cure. I did have feelings of anger, resentment and was depressed when I realized that the pain was not temporary. I finally coped by evaluating the changes in my lifestyle as I learned to accept that permanent pain and varying levels of disability were part of my new reality.

---

[15] 7 Stages of Greif, Through the Process and Back to Life, recover-from-grief.com

Family and friends who form the support group around the patient must be educated and aware of the fluid nature of RSD. Fluid meaning that symptoms come and go, the patient might be up one minute and down the next, have a fever, sweating, swelling, discoloration and the like and then it settles down until the next flare-up. If the caretakers learn the possible treatment and rehabilitation options, patient's behaviors that should be encouraged or discouraged, and take the supporting role, the family and patient will better communicate with each other. It is very important for friends and family to try to understand what the patient is going through and allow the patient the opportunity to express his or her emotions. Patients need to feel that they can show their grief and frustration without being judged by their supporters. I am lucky to have family and friends who are supportive and encourage me to keep my spirits up and to continue functioning to the best of my ability.

Not all treatments work for all RSD patients. Pushing different treatment modalities is harmful to the communication process. Like me, patients get tired of being "lab rats." Although making suggestions is a positive behavior for a family member or friend, do not get discouraged as a supporter if the patient chooses something else or had tried what you suggested and it did not work for them.

Some patients become depressed if their condition prevents them from doing things that are important to their independence and well-being. I was an independent person who had to learn how to rely on others for daily tasks (e.g., dressing, cooking, and errands). This is not only inconvenient, but can lead to feeling worthless and can be demeaning. Having independence taken away tends to rob patients of their self-respect. It is important to address these feelings and to respond appropriately as a supporter. Attitude and self-perception are crucial factors for continuing to maintain a good quality of life. As patients struggle with their situation, they may be having feelings of inadequacy and worthlessness. You can encourage them to be social and participate in life activities through positive communication. Patients may find benefit in some of the following activities:

- Counseling, or having someone to talk to other than their caretakers
- Exercising at the appropriate levels

- Getting involved with a spiritual group
- Keeping a journal
- Reading, watching movies or TV
- Setting goals (e.g., daily, weekly, monthly)
- Volunteering

From my experiences, I would suggest that a patient be encouraged to join a support group or to seek psychological counseling, if appropriate. Be sure to find a support group that focuses on a positive patient life and social skills. Patients may even reach the point of mentoring and counseling others with RSD. Some patients find benefit in getting involved in volunteer work. Volunteering allows them to set their own hours and to feel that they can still contribute to others instead of just focusing on their own condition.

Despite a wide range of treatment options available to patients with RSD, some patients do not seek help. Patients may be discouraged from reaching out by constant pain. They are worn down both physically and emotionally. This may result in dismissing support and effort from others to help them. Some patients are concerned with fears. Fear that nothing can help them or that the side effects from treatments will be too much to handle. They fear that they will become addicted to the medications or they will develop a tolerance to medications and the recurring pain will be even worse. Patients often hear that they are seen as "complainers" if they talk about their pain, so a fear of communication can develop.

It is important for the patient to discuss these concerns with family members, friends, physicians, and support service professionals (e.g., psychologist, social worker) in order to take advantage of options that are available. These options may actually lead to pain relief and improvement in the overall quality of their life. Helping them through the fear makes the whole process easier on them.

WORK: THE OUTSIDE CONNECTION

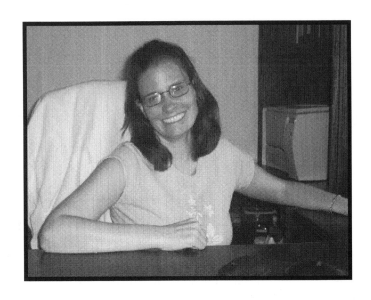

With chronic pain, just getting dressed in the morning is an ordeal. Add to that the prospect of a commute to the office, long hours spent sitting at a desk and the commute home. It is exhausting for me to just think about. Walking more than a block or two would wear me down before the start of the day. But there are other options. I was able to work from home for an attorney. I ordered medical records and organized case files for personal injury cases. I could do it at my own speed and when I was feeling okay to work with full concentration. It is all right to work part of the day, rest and go back to work. On days that the pain is unbearable, I just did not work at all. Working this way allowed me to deal with my health. I spent approximately five hours a week, and it was a great job for me. This type of work has emerged as a viable alternative for many companies. For the chronically disabled, the "work from home" industry has made life easier for many of us. It is invaluable for people who can work, just not from a corporate office or having set hours. Many employers are using this approach with able-bodied workers as well. Companies that allow employees to work from home can help companies retain talent and keep the brightest people with their companies. In December 1999, Congress created the Work Incentives Improvement Act and the Ticket to Work program through our Social Security System. These programs allow for people with disabilities to reintegrate into the workforce easier. The programs provide better healthcare coverage, increased choice of rehab, and employment services for workers with disabilities. The WIIA laws help people who are planning to work or are working with disabilities already. The act was designed to have work programs to keep pace with medical advances, assistive technologies, and the changing dynamics of the new workplace.[16] The WIIA and the Ticket to Work program, in combination with the work from home jobs available, encourages and allows disability beneficiaries to return to work.

If you decide to return to work, you will need to decide when and how to disclose your disability. It is a good idea to speak with your doctor when considering returning to work. Let him know your concerns. Find out what the doctor thinks about your functional capabilities related to the type of work you are trying to pursue. Is there any durable medical equipment that may assist you in taking a job, and can the doctor write a prescription for the equipment? Finally, find out what he thinks about your prognosis and limitations. Let the human resources person you interview with know up front about "set-in-stone" limitations or needs.

Once you are able to work, you will go through some sort of interviewing process. This can be very intimidating and stressful. When approached with a plan, your chances of a successful hiring are greater. In an

---

[16] Ticket to Work and Work Incentives Improvement Act of 1999, Public Law 106-170

interview, be concise. Say something like, "For the last three years, I've been dealing with a medical issue, but it's under control now." Do not overlook the skills you have developed as a result of living with an invisible disability. You can say something like, "creative problem solving, flexibility and determination have been skills I was able to improve when learning to deal with my disability." You can emphasize your coping strategies by staying positive.

According to the American Pain Foundation, over 76,000,000 people have chronic pain and 25,000,000 more have acute pain; that is about one in four Americans who live with pain every day. Remember that anyone can develop a disability, invisible or not, at any time, and the interviewer may know someone in a similar situation. Do not automatically assume that this is the case. You can mention your disability when the other person says, "Tell me about yourself." Take this opportunity to talk about your disability briefly, clearly and without being defensive. It is a good time to also tell the person about any accommodations or coping strategies you have developed as a result of your disability to reinforce the proactive steps you have taken and to show them that despite your disability, you are a positive and productive person.

SEXUALITY AND INTIMACY ISSUES

NOTE: If you think that your sex drive is not normal due to a side effect of a medication you are taking, it is important to speak to your doctor about it. Medications can also cause a lack in libido.

Intimacy is an important aspect in keeping a healthy lifestyle. Often times, chronic pain patients forget that sexuality is an important part in a partnered relationship when their pain levels are high. In spite of chronic pain, you and your significant other can have an active sexual relationship that is quite satisfying. You just have to be creative with getting around the challenges of chronic pain. All people need emotional and physical intimacy. The vital need for human connection helps stimulate our sexuality. Sex is an important aspect of our identity, and when chronic pain comes into the picture, it is often the last thing we are concerned with nurturing.

Talking with your partner is the first step in reclaiming your sexuality. Try starting the discussion fully clothed, in the living room or in a neutral setting. When speaking, use "I" so that you're not putting stress, pressure or anxiety on your partner. An example is, "I love when you hold me close; it makes me feel cared for" versus "You must not love me; you never touch me." Maybe the partner is afraid of causing you pain, and if you let him or her know you are still interested and willing to have intimacy, you can put your partner at ease. Conclusions you may have jumped to as to why your partner has stopped touching you can be cleared up. It is usually not that they lost interest in sex or in you or that they now find you undesirable.

When trying to raise the love and intimacy between the two of you, try doing things that will make the other feel loved and appreciated. Start with emotional intimacy: let them know that you are attracted to them, that you appreciate all they do for you and that you are open to their affections. Learn more about what makes your partner feel good, and reconnect with an exploration of each other's bodies, not specifically for orgasm, but a sense of learning about each other all over again.

If you are having trouble with spontaneity, make a date for sex in advance. Pick a time of day when you have the most energy and least pain, and tell your partner, "This is our intimate time." Make sure to incorporate time to try new things. Staying relaxed and focusing on the pleasure as it happens will help you move along. There may also be a need for humor. For instance, if you suddenly feel you want to get into a new position and as soon as you get into it you realize you are going to fall over or you turn into a pretzel just trying to get into the position. When this happens, get back to focusing on the great experience and return to a position you know you both will enjoy. The bottom line is keep going, you can rest afterwards. You may also find that you feel better after sex. During sex, endorphins build up and are released during orgasm. Endorphins are the body's natural painkillers, so take advantage of them.

Chronic pain can cause an emotional wedge between you and your partner. Becoming aware that your physical and emotional distance hurts your partner may add to your fear, guilt, resentment and anxiety. Relationship problems can exacerbate stress even in strong relationships. Medical problems like chronic pain lead to unemployment, financial issues, a less kept house and lower self-esteem that can uncover previously hidden conflicts with your partner. If you do not have a plan, you may suffer in the human connection and intimacy area.

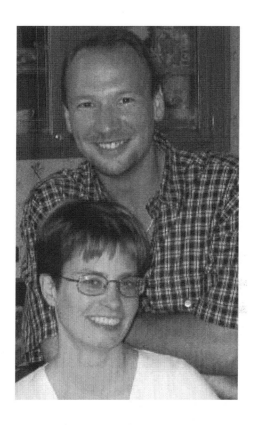

If you are feeling unattractive and undesirable, your own actions may be preventing the intimacy you desire. Become aware of your needs and your partner's needs for sexual contact and passion. There are times when sex seems out of the question. There are times when I am simply hurting too much or feel too tired for sex. However, I will try to remember that my partner needs the love just as much as I do and that for this period of time, I can get my mind off of the pain. When I am planning for intimacy ahead of time, I can take stronger pain control medication so that I can experience the same pleasure my partner is feeling. Also, medications can lower your libido just as a low self-esteem does. Some medications lower sex drive by affecting blood flow and hormones. The want for sex is also diminished by changes in your nervous system. Keeping this in mind will help your plan stay in effect and increase the satisfaction of your partner and your own intimate needs.

Intimacy is explored through petting, masturbation, sexual intercourse, exploring your partner, oral sex, different positions, sex toys, and lubricants. Having actual intercourse is just one way to create closeness. Being creative is a way to enhance and amplify your intimacy needs. Things such as holding hands, cuddling, fondling, massaging and kissing increase these intimacy feelings. If you are unable to be very active, your partner may use masturbation during mutual sexual activity. Also oral sex can be an alternative to traditional intercourse. Keep in mind that many medications cause a problem with natural lubricant processing. This problem can be solved with over-the-counter lubricants and help prevent pain associated with vaginal dryness. There are books at the library, online and in bookstores that can be used as guides to creative intercourse. The bottom line is that intimacy and sexuality can actually make you feel better. The sexual contact you achieve while having sex can help you feel stronger and the intimacy you build with your partner will help you both better cope with your chronic pain.

SUICIDE AND SPIRITUALITY WITH PAIN

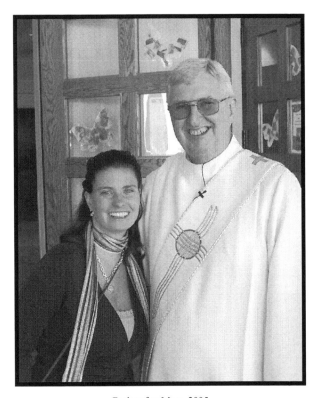

Barby after Mass, 2005

Because currently there is no cure for RSD, the disorder may persist for a prolonged period of time and can have a significant psychosocial impact on patients. The chronic, severe nature of pain experienced by many RSD patients, particularly those with established and long-

142

standing RSD, may lead to psychological co-morbidity, including anxiety, feelings of isolation, depression, and a sense of hopelessness and helplessness. In some cases, the adverse psychological consequences of the RSD may increase the risk of suicide or suicide ideation. It is, therefore, important for patients and their families to recognize and understand the potential psychological effects of RSD and seek a thorough psychological consultation and evaluation as part of the overall strategy for managing RSD.

A variety of different treatment options are available to help RSD patients with concurrent psychological co-morbidity, including drug therapy and cognitive behavior therapy. A multidisciplinary approach to treatment involving a pain management specialist, neurologist, physiatrist (specialist in physical medicine and rehabilitation), and a psychologist or psychiatrist may be necessary to help RSD patients learn to better cope and adjust to both the physical and psychological consequences of the disorder.

Your attitude and self-perception are crucial factors for continuing to maintain a good life. As I struggle with my situation with sometimes, feelings of inadequacy and worthlessness, I find it beneficial to keep a journal, set realistic goals, attend church, learn and read. I use these tools to increase my knowledge of myself as well as gain useful knowledge about the RSD in me and to grow stronger spiritually.

All humans experience pain. Like me, many people spend time trying to find something in our spirituality that offers an escape from our pain. Pain is part of our reality, humanity and responsibility. Understanding that not all pain is bad is important in this process. As humans, we need pain to keep us from danger and lead us to responsible activities that prolong our race and ourselves. Chronic pain is bad pain. Pain becomes bad when it outstays its usefulness. When you have bad pain, it is just that: bad pain. Trying to ignore it is harmful to us and to society. Bad pain must be dealt with as it affects our spirituality and our willingness to carry on humanity and our responsibility to God. Often we ask ourselves, "Is somehow having chronic pain a way for God to test my strength?"

Pain is often associated with suffering. Does our suffering improve our ability to help humanity? At one point or another, my pain has affected my creativity and has caused chaos when not put into perspective. Many people make a choice to move closer to God or close Him out when a chronic condition affects them directly. For me, I have found a deeper awareness of God's presence in my life and in those around me. I choose to look at the world through positivism and miracles. There are dark times in most chronic pain sufferers' paths where we contemplate what we are here for. Finding a goal and the path to follow is important to keeping up our spirits. Without goals and direction, we tend to create disharmony and chaos. If we are not aware of God in our life, our pain loses its humanity. To stop LIVING would be the worst thing we could do to get through the pain. Turning to our higher power and using our worldly tools will help us achieve for the greater good of everyone.

Through physical activity, we LIVE and pick up our spirits. Remembering to keep within my appropriate level of exercising or physical movement, every now and then, I push myself a little beyond to see if I have made any gains. I usually end up paying for it the next few days, but I am glad to have made it through the test and know where my new boundaries lie. My spirituality has really come into play with my physical abilities as well. Many days and nights, I pray that I will make it through another successful activity. I believe the saying, "God only gives you what you can handle." However, I also wish He did not think I could handle so much. The fact that I am LIVING and handling the pain is a testament to my faith and my abilities I did not know I had.

Pain is ultimately a mystery to us all. Sometimes nothing can be done about the causes of chronic pain in our life. When I have no choices and am only pain-filled, believing that we are the body of Christ and the final glory will be in all, the pain becomes more bearable for me. My suffering leads to the suffering of all involved in my life. It takes a toll on all of us because of our inability to know what to do.

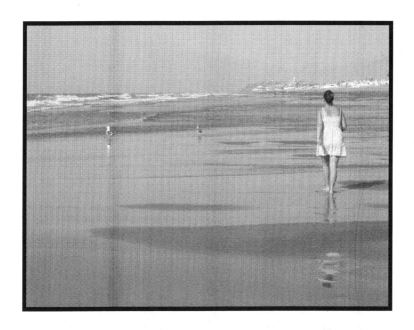

When I am in severe pain, I try to share the pain experience with others, not to complain, but to find understanding, despite knowing deep down that we can never feel what someone else's pain is like. As we encounter pain, we become stronger in faith or weaker in faith. Pain can destroy a person and those around him. If you allow it, pain will destroy everything good in your life. Those of us who live a life of unsought pain represent the mystery of life and our deep need for survival as a race. My spirituality has grown from my need for survival. My daily prayer and hope is to lessen the pain. As the pain transforms me, my instinct for survival, which is a deep instinct for us all, strengthens me and helps me stay in the light of God's grace.

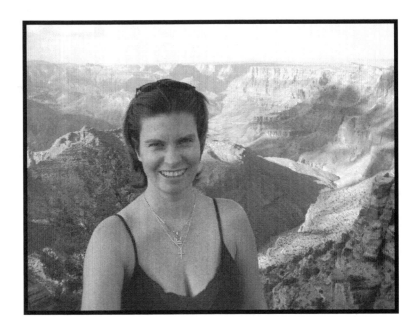

RECAP

- All humans experience pain.

- Believing we are the Body of Christ and that final glory will be in all, pain becomes more bearable for me.

- Many people make a choice to move closer to or shut out God when a chronic condition affects them directly.

- Our spirituality can offer an escape from our pain.

- Pain affects creativity and causes chaos when not put into proper perspective.

- Pain is part of reality, humanity and responsibility.

- There are dark times in most chronic pain sufferers' paths where we contemplate what we are here for.

- To stop LIVING would be the worst thing we could do to get through the pain and to honor GOD.

CHILDREN WITH RSD

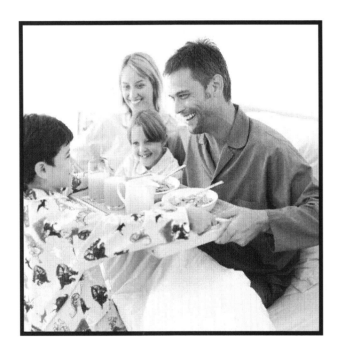

It is usually shocking and unexpected when you learn that your child has a chronic pain illness and that it can last a lifetime. Parents often feel a sense of devastation, powerlessness, uncertainty of where to turn, and uncertainty for your child's future. Many adults with RSD have trouble coping; it seems cruel to have to watch a child go through this awful condition. I was an adult (29) when I developed RSD so, I am writing this without the personal experience of childhood chronic illness. Unfortunately, anyone at any age can get RSD. The good news for children is that studies show that they are more likely to go into remission than adults with RSD. I have spoken with both RSD children and their parents about their experience, about what to expect and coping skills they have learned. I have learned a few things from them that I am passing on.

First, a child will feel more supported and loved if you educate yourself about what they are going through. Secondly, helping your child through the stresses of life is something good parents do already. Chronic illness patients deal with more stress than healthy people. Taking on the issue of stress reduction in your life and theirs is important. With RSD, your child will go through adult situations. They will have to cope with many doctor visits, hospital visits, painful procedures, imperfect body, loss of mobility, loss of social activity, loss of friends, and even a possibility of premature death. These are all tough issues for even the most mature of adults. Helping your children through predictable periods of stress can be done by creating a plan and keeping to a routine. Children will go through predictable fears and anxieties with each approaching procedure and may feel more apprehensive and unsafe if they see that your reaction is also full of fear. Children watch how you react to a situation or bad news and can take on your stress. The more you speak to your child about their illness, the more they will be comfortable and open about expressing their needs and emotional state, and the less stress and anxiety they will carry. Let the child know that they are not going through this physical pain because of disobeying you, and it is not a punishment for something they did. There is no simple way to help your child avoid stressful medical situations, but there are a few suggestions to assist with the situations as they arise.

Be sure to use age appropriate terms and prepare them for what is coming up in the immediate future. You do not need to let them know the whole plan of treatment at once; it can be overwhelming for them and cause undue stress and anxiety. When having these conversations emphasize their strength while dealing with the situation. Gauge what you tell them by the types of questions they are asking. Toddlers and young children need very general concepts, as that is all they can conceive. As children grow up they can better understand the technical information, be part of bigger decision-making and eventually assume responsibility for their own care. Children typically will give you signals, as they are ready to assume great responsibility. When your child is avoiding the move to greater independence check your behavior. Are you teaching your child to perform certain tasks even though they are disabled or are you giving them too much special attention?

Talk to them prior to appointments, and let them know what they will be facing at the doctor, upcoming procedures and hospital stays. Ask them if there is anything you can do to help them. For instance, when getting a shot, do they want you to hold their hand or give them their favorite teddy bear to hold? Asking them simple questions while the needle is being inserted is also a useful distraction from the stress of the situation. Children tend to be afraid of the unknown. If you are able to have other children who are going through similar treatments speak with your child, they might have some great tips. You can always ask your doctor for a referral to other patients and their parents going through similar circumstances. You can help your child become familiar with the surroundings of the doctor office or hospital setting by going early to walk them around the area. This gets the child familiar with their surroundings, and they may feel like there is less uncertainty with the situation. Children tend to be afraid of the unknown. Let your child choose how to control their situation when possible. For example, give them the option of when the procedure will occur (Monday or Wednesday), which arm they want the IV inserted into, or what reward they will get for following the doctors and nurses directions.

Children should be able to communicate to you their frustration, rage, sadness and stress without fear of you becoming upset. Being open and honest with your child lowers anxiety levels, and they gain a greater respect and trust in you, their caretaker. Children count on you to protect them. You have to be their advocate with the healthcare world, the school system and all social settings. If they feel that you will not stand up for them or with them, their behavior may turn negative more easily and more often. You can remind them of what they can do well despite the condition and that you are proud that they are trying hard to get through a rough situation. Try to not become a hostage to RSD. Keep in mind that just because the child is in pain does not mean it is always a level ten.

Take advantage of their lower pain level times by planning fun and interesting activities that offer a rewarding experience. Even mastering activities of daily living can raise a child's self-esteem and pride. You can do a refresher with your kids, each year on RSD. You both may be reminded of a tip or tool you can use to make everyday life better. Also, new treatments and medications are becoming available. Don't get stuck in what was available when the RSD first came on. Keep up your knowledge and education; fill in gaps and misconceptions in your child's view of the disorder. And show a continued hope for better treatments in the future. Coming to terms with your child's condition will enable your child to do the same.

Take time to praise yourself for dealing with your child's RSD. As a parent you will also have to deal with your feelings of anger, rage and sadness. There will be times when you are resentful and worried about their future. Having the wisdom and courage to take control of the situation will make you stronger. Remember, even parents of healthy children have their moments of resentment, doubt, anxiety and fear. Putting life into perspective and taking on challenges with a positive outlook will help both you and your child.

TIPS

- As your child grows, include them more in creating and finalizing the next treatment plan.

- Children with RSD are usually healthy, they just happen to have a chronic pain condition.

- Develop some guidelines for sensible restrictions.

- Discuss your concerns with your child's doctor.

- Encouraging your child to participate in social activities.

- Knowledge is power: try to stay educated & up-to-date about new treatments and coping tools.

- Update your plan, at least yearly.

- While RSD may creates difficulties for children, with the support of their parents, they can lead effective, exciting lives & grow to become productive adults.

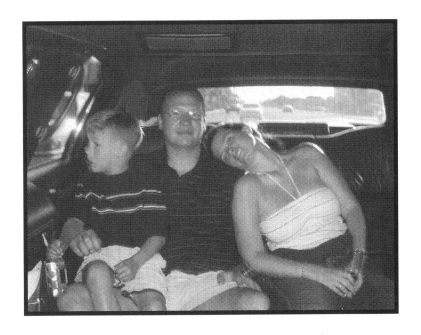

When the patient is the parent, it is important to include the children (whether they are your own, nephews/nieces or grandkids) whenever possible. Teach the children to be as self-sufficient as possible when they are around you. Help them see it is a positive thing that they are able to do things on their own, like make their own bowl of cereal or carry their dirty laundry to the laundry room. Help them see that disabled people can lead active lives by emphasizing the things you can do, rather than what you can't do. Praising children for their help will give them a sense of pride, and they will be more eager to assist next time help is needed. It is important that kids can look at the person the same way they would with any other person in the family.

As a patient, let your family knows it is all right to ask questions. Many people think asking someone about their disability is offensive. It is quite the contrary: when you are dealing with a newly disabled person in the family or with anyone disabled for the first time, it is natural to be curious. The same is true for the disabled person. Asking questions is usually acceptable, as long as you use common sense. Find out what equipment or techniques are needed to do activities of daily living and how they will get around and how their medications or tens unit works. If you are able, offer your assistance when necessary.

Although some disabled people are unwilling to accept help, it is usually appropriate to lend a hand if they are having obvious difficulty. If they are giving you a hard time, try relating your assistance to pulling over and offering assistance to a motorist with a flat tire. By offering to give assistance, you did your part, so the disabled person should be willing to take what you are offering. For some, it is very difficult to take help after leading a self-reliant life. As time passes, they may become more accepting of help.

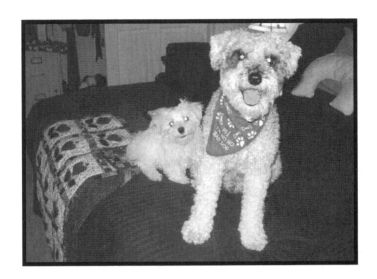

We all have obstacles to overcome no matter who we are. When you are a healthy person faced with a challenge, think about how you feel when others want to help you. What if you are heavy set, bald or short and people are treating you differently from the rest of the family. Like you, the disabled person would rather not be pitied or shunned because of their disability. They would much rather be accepted for who they are. Recognizing that the disabled person in the family has normal thoughts and feelings can go a long way. Just by asking questions, offering assistance, and putting yourself in their shoes can help all of your lives in a positive, healthy way, and you might learn more about yourself in the process.

If you are the spouse of a pain patient and you have children, you may worry about the effect of the pain on them. Be sure to include your children. Children often grieve that the new disability is something they caused or something they can cure. My nephew came to visit and I was having a bad day. He asked his mother if he could give me some hot chocolate and cookies to make me feel better. She did not know how to explain to him that this condition was permanent and, although I appreciate the gesture, I am going to always need some assistance and may not always feel good.

RECAP

- Children may also get depressed about the loss of attention and affection from you as a caretaker and the parent in pain.

- Children may be upset from the loss of activities due to financial limitations.

- Children may blame themselves.

- When the parent's is the one in pain, it is important to let the children know that it is not their fault.

LIVING WITH BODY WIDE RSD

It is hard to imagine your whole body in burning pain or, as some BW-RSD'ers describe it, standing in a swarm of mad bees that do not die. Not just your arm, shoulder, neck, face and foot, but the burn continues in every part of your body. It is in your head, stomach, feet, muscles, skin and just about every other part. For a number of RSD patients, RSD does go body wide. For these unlucky people the pain travels indiscriminately through your body.

Treatments for patients with body wide RSD are not different from someone with it in one to three limbs. The difference comes in with how quickly you tire, how much physical activity you can perform, and how much physical touching you can handle. Getting a handle on what aspects of your behavior lead to increased pain levels, setting up a strong support system, and staying positive will all help in this overwhelming battle. Patients who have RSD body wide also have similar stories to those with only one extremity affected. They have had multiple surgeries or injuries over a period of at least a few years. As they got worse, doctors were unable to find any reason for the additional pain or spreading that was occurring. As a result of going doctor to doctor, looking for some kind of answer, patients encounter doctors who don't understand why RSD spreads, or if they are performing the wrong treatments, and these doctors actually contributed to the problems. Dealing with body wide RSD also plays more severe emotional aspects if not confronted and worked through.

Going through test after test and procedure after procedure, a diagnosis of RSD is finally given. This is partially due to the fact that other conditions needed to be ruled out prior to RSD diagnosis. The pain usually starts from the original injury and spreads over time to other body parts. With each level of progression, the pain becomes less tolerable, social interaction diminishes, and life changes become more permanent. Many body wide patients have or have had pain pumps and spinal cord stimulators. They are on maximum doses of narcotics. The invasive measures often have to have follow-up surgeries due to complications such as infections or battery-life of the medical equipment implanted. Each additional insult or trauma to the body poses a greater risk of swelling. This is how desperate RSD'ers have become. We are willing to go through risky procedures and have foreign objects implanted that can cause the RSD to worsen, as if your pain can't get worse when it is already a ten on the pain scale.

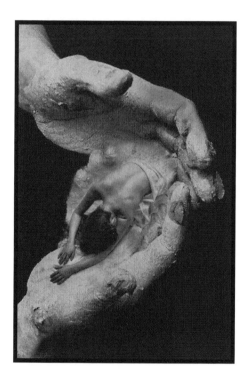

Actually, I rated the pain I had in the beginning a ten. I did not think I could take anything worse. As each surgery or procedure was performed and the pain worsened, I realized that I wish I had that first pain back if I

164

had to have pain at all. As our bodies get "used to the pain", the pain is easier to manage and deal with. With each additional trauma or spread of the RSD, the pain you thought was unbearable becomes an okay level. Unfortunately, the pain causes our personalities to change and affects the family and friends around us. Most people will never truly understand the physical pain and emotional pain RSD patients endure. They will never know how strong you have to be to deal with such life changing issues. Finding something to give you purpose can be your saving grace. Taking a job from home, volunteering for an organization or finding someone to mentor can be done if you are upfront from the start and let the people know that you have good days and moments and at times you may have to back out of things. I need extra time when given a project to accomplish and that can become overwhelming for me. Making sure the person I am working with understands ahead of time helps keep the lines of communication open.

Along with the extreme physical pain of body wide RSD, it affects many other facets of a patient's life. The extreme changes in your social life, the loss of physical relationships, and the fight against depression are constant struggles. You can live through it and you can have a greater purpose in life. Life is not over until you die or choose not to LIVE. There are times I feel like I am going to die from this pain, but I don't; I get through it. I have learned to turn to prayer and believe that I deep down want to do my damndest to live my life as much as I am able to on my own. If you are unable to get out, you can find others going through similar struggles through the Internet. If you don't have a computer, you can always call RSDHope and be paired through their mentor program to speak with other patients by phone. Learn through trial and error, get involved, and have a greater reason to get out of bed. Concentrate on the great things in your life rather than the pain and negative situation you have to deal with. How you look at life will change how you live your life. As we fight and speak out and as long as there are others like us, we can choose to LIVE. Letting others know they are not alone helps them and can in turn help you.

OUR FUTURE

To make informed and wise decisions about your treatment plan, doctors, hospitals and taking your life back from the pain in you, become educated. This book series is one step in the education process. Places to look for additional Information that is up-to-date with RSD issues are:

- Clinical trials and Studies
- Disease organizations
- Internet health sites
- Support groups for RSD or Chronic Pain

The important part for you is sorting through all of the information that you do gather so that it can be processed in terms that you, your family and doctors will all understand to make informed decisions. When the need for more advanced information still exists, you need to dig deeper. For instance, knowing the experts and best locations for medical treatment of RSD patients is necessary. Going further, you should follow those experts

167

as they publish new findings. You never know when the miracle is going to happen. Until then, use the tools available to you from many sources. This way you will get the best and most accurate information to deal with your specific issues.

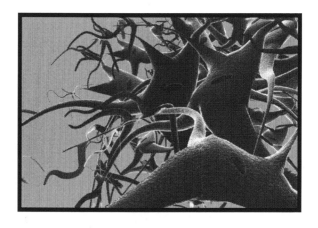

Reduction in small-fiber nerves may underlie complex regional pain syndrome-I (reflex sympathetic dystrophy). Researchers at Massachusetts General Hospital (MGH) have found the first pieces of evidence of a physical abnormality underlying the chronic pain condition called reflex sympathetic dystrophy (RSD) or complex regional pain syndrome-I (CRPS-I). In the February issue of their journal, Pain, they describe finding that skin affected by CRPS-I pain appears to have lost some small-fiber nerve endings, a change that is characteristic of other neuropathic pain syndromes. "This sort of small-fiber degeneration has been found in every nerve pain condition ever studied, including post-herpetic neuralgia and neuropathies associated with diabetes and HIV infection," says Anne Louise Oaklander, MD, PhD. "The nerve damage in those conditions has been much more severe, which may be why it's been so hard to detect CRPS-I-related nerve damage." [17]

Because small-fiber nerve endings transmit pain messages and control skin color and temperature and because damage to those fibers is associated with other painful disorders, the MGH research team hypothesized that those fibers might also be involved with CRPS-I. To investigate their theory, they studied 18 CRPS-I patients and seven control patients with similar chronic symptoms known to be caused by arthritis. Small skin biopsies were taken under anesthesia from the most painful area, from a pain-free area on the same limb and from a corresponding unaffected area on the other side of the body.

---

[17] Anne Louise Oaklander, M.D., Ph.D., director of Massachusetts General Hospital Nerve Unit, lead the study on Small Nerve Fiber and RSD.

TIPS

- Continue to research and keep a positive attitude that relief is possible.

- Follow RSD experts as they publish new findings

- Get your information organized.

- Make informed and wise decisions about your treatment plan, doctors, best hospitals for you, and taking your life back from the pain in you, you have to become educated.

- Massachusetts General Hospital staff has found the first evidence of a physical abnormality underlying RSD.

- There is hope for treatments of RSD that are putting patients into remission: new research results and procedures are coming that will assist in patient care on a long-term basis.

SECTION THREE

MANAGING YOUR RSD
IN THE HEALTHCARE INDUSTRY

TIPS FOR FINDING PHYSICIANS

Finding a highly qualified, competent, and compassionate physician to manage your specific illness or condition takes a lot of hard work and energy, but it is an investment that is well worth the effort. I have met over 90 healthcare providers, including hospital staff, neurologists, cardiologists, psychologists, X-ray technicians, pain management, general practice, orthopedic and the list goes on. It is important to keep in mind that you are not looking for just any general physician but rather a physician who has expertise in the treatment and management of your specific illness or condition. Find out if the doctor knows about RSD in-depth. Sometimes a pain doctor will know more about arthritis then neuropathy pain because of the types of classes taken in medical school and previous patients. It does not make him or her a bad doctor, just not necessarily the right one for you.

It has generally been assumed by many people that the longer a physician has been in practice, the more experience, knowledge, and skills they have accumulated and, therefore, the higher the quality of care they provide to their patients. Recent research conducted by a group of doctors from the Harvard Medical School, however, seems to strongly suggest that this premise may not be true. In an article published in February 2005 in the Annals of Internal Medicine, the Harvard researchers seriously challenged the common assumption that the more clinical experience a physician has accumulated, the higher the level of medical care they provide to their patients.

In fact, surprisingly, the researchers found an inverse (opposite) relationship between the number of years that a physician has been in practice (i.e., experience) and the quality of care that the physician provides. In other words, the widely held belief that "practice makes perfect" does not necessarily apply to all physicians and should not be the sole criteria used by patients in their decision analysis for choosing a physician. The underlying message of this study is that the length of time a physician has been in practice does not necessarily equate to a high quality of medical care unless the doctor takes steps to keep abreast with new advances and changing patterns of clinical practice.[18]

---

[18] Annals of Internal Medicine, Vol 142.4. 260-303

There are some important issues you need to consider and carefully research before making an informed decision about choosing your doctor. Find out whether they are board certified, medical school affiliations, hospital associations, and the hospital's accreditations. Board certified means that the doctor is required to have extra training after medical school to become a specialist in a particular field of medicine and are required to take continuing education courses in order to maintain their board certification status. You can check to see if a doctor is board certified in each state through the medical board of your state. In Arizona, it is easy to check because they have an online site. You can also check with the American Board of Medical Specialists (ABMS) to determine if a specific physician you are considering is board certified in a particular medical specialty. Next, find out if the doctor you are considering also has a joint faculty appointment at a medical school. In general, practicing community physicians with a joint academic appointment at a medical school are more likely to be in contact with leading medical experts and may be more up-to-date with the latest advances in research and treatments than community-based physicians who are not affiliated with a medical school.

Then, research to find out about the hospitals that the doctor uses. In the event that you need to be treated at a hospital, is the hospital where the physician has admitting privileges near your home or will you (and your family members) have to travel a considerable distance? It is also a good idea to find out if the Joint Commission on Accreditation of Healthcare Organizations (JCAHO) accredits the hospital where the physician has admitting privileges.[19] You can find information about a specific hospital's accreditation status by searching the JCAHO Internet site.

The JCAHO is an independent, not-for-profit organization that evaluates and accredits more than 15,000 healthcare organizations and programs in the United States. To receive and maintain JCAHO accreditation, a healthcare organization must undergo an on-site survey by a JCAHO survey team at least every three years and meet specific standards and performance measurements that affect the safety and quality of patient care. Finally, as noted above, remember that how long a physician has been in practice (i.e., experience) does not necessarily correlate with a high level of medical expertise you will need with RSD.

---

[19] Joint Commission on Accreditation of Healthcare Organizations (JCAHO)

PREPARING FOR DOCTOR VISITS

Learning to communicate with your healthcare professionals is important in your treatment plan. Increasing your communication leads to better treatment and pain relief. Better communication starts with organization.

TIPS

- Be assertive and listen to the other side.
- Become the expert of your pain.
- Have a shared understanding of goals.
- Start a pain journal.
- Take responsibility to reach the goals.
- Take someone with you.
- Write your questions; take notes.

When preparing to see a doctor you should get organized. Start with a review of past treatments for pain. Ask yourself, "Are they working, and what makes the pain better or worse?" It is good to keep a journal on your activities and pain levels so that you can reflect on these questions. Prepare a personal history, be brief, and stick to the needed information. If there are any concerns about your medications or if you would like to try a different medication you have researched, be able to explain why to your doctor. Finally, get your emotions under control. I have found that if you go into the office showing frustration, anger, anxiety or other negatively perceived emotions, the doctors are less likely to be able to provide you with useful tools. They will focus on your mental status first, which is not always bad. If you need help with pain or an infection, letting your emotions get the best of you at the doctors office will create trouble succeeding if further treatment is your ultimate goal. If you prepare ahead of time, you may have these emotions, but you will be able to handle them better as they arise. You will also have a more productive doctor visit by staying on track and progressing forward with a plan set by you and your healthcare provider.

I have experienced this phenomenon a lot in the beginning of my search for proper treatment and diagnosis. After so many doctors who say, "Do you want to get better? It is all in your head, so I can't help you. Try a different doctor. I am stumped, and these symptoms don't make sense," go into the appointment having evaluated yourself and your symptoms. Keep yourself in check, stay calm and positive, and assist the doctor with finding the answers so that the outcome will be more beneficial for you at the appointment and in the end.

DURING YOUR MEDICAL VISIT

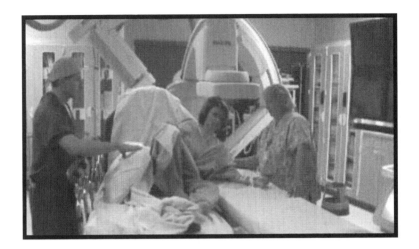

It is important that you stay on track and focused at your doctor appointments. The more you are prepared and on track the better your care will be. It is also important to keep your emotions under control. Therefore, in a positive controlled manner convey the following:

- Are there any new options for non-drug pain control methods?
- Describe what your pain feels like: burning, cutting, stabbing, deep, tingling, etc. Different types of pain can be treated with different medications. Be as

179

descriptive as possible for a better outcome with pain relief.

- Express what makes pain better/worse - it helps to keep a journal.

- How does the pain affect your daily living: do you need help dressing, bathing, or cooking?

- Show where it hurts: point to the areas; if it is your whole body, does any part hurt more than the rest or does the pain feel different in different spots?

- State what concerns or worries you have regarding the pain, medications; e.g., What if the pain just doesn't go away?

- What has happened to you medically since your last visit?

Put all of this information into a summary so that you stay on track and the doctor gets all of the needed information. Leave the sheet with the doctor to put in your records, so if something comes up he can refer to it and better remember what you may need if an emergency comes up. Keep in mind that doctors have hundreds to thousands of patients, so they sometimes need reminders. It does not mean that they do not care about you. Taking control of your healthcare team will facilitate communication, better treatment, and quality pain care assistance. Be sure that you are keeping all of your healthcare providers abreast of your condition, goals, progress and setbacks. This team includes all doctors (primary, neurologist, pain management and other specialties), physical therapists and caregivers.

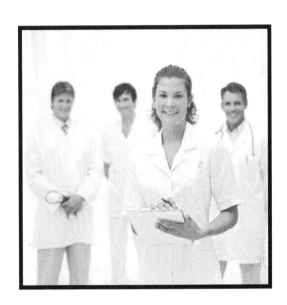

EXAMPLE OF NOTES TO BRING TO DOCTOR VISITS

Suzie Badhealth, 1/22/06

Medication

- List Current Medications w/ dosages
- List of any past medications w/ bad reactions

Recent Issues

- New Medication: Neurotin- Started Neurotin on 1/10/06 @ 300 mg (night) wk 1, (then move to - 300 mg (M & N) wk 2, - 300 mg (M, N & N)

Recent Tests/procedure

- Radio Frequency Treatment- January 13, 2006

Continuing Issues

- RSD- Pain (Arm, fingers, shoulder, neck, face, foot), Eyegraines, migraines, dizziness, memory, vision hearing, balance/falls.
- Weight Loss

Questions

- Are there any known long term effects from the Radio Frequency Ablations?

Past Surgeries

- 1999- Hysterectomy, Endometriosis, 2001- Right Knee Surgery, Torn Meniscus and MCL, 2003- Right Rib Resection, Thoracic Outlet Syndrome

Given to: Dr. Rubin, Dr. Hummel, Date Given: 1/22/2006

WORKING WITH YOUR DOCTORS

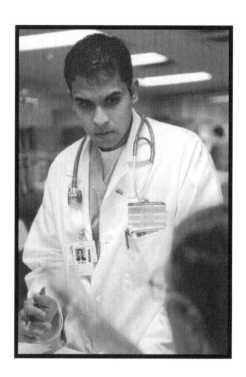

One of the most important decisions confronting patients who have been diagnosed with a serious medical condition is choosing a qualified physician who will deliver a high level and quality of medical care in accordance with currently accepted guidelines and standards of care. Finding the "best" doctor to manage your condition, however, can be a frustrating and a time-consuming

183

experience unless you know what you are looking for and how to go about finding it. In the beginning of my ordeal, I followed what the doctors told me to the letter, even when I had doubts about the recommendation. My focus was on getting better, and I was brought up to believe that doctors knew better that "regular people." They always know what to do and have all the answers. It took me almost three years after my accident to realize that this was a complete myth. Healthcare providers are human too, and they can make mistakes.

The process of finding and choosing a physician to manage your specific illness or condition is, in some respects, comparable to the process of making a decision about whether or not to invest in a particular stock or mutual fund. After all, you would not invest your hard-earned money in a stock without first doing exhaustive research about the stock's past performance, current financial status, and projected future earnings. More than likely you would spend a considerable amount of time and energy doing your own research and consulting with your stockbroker before making a decision about investing. The same general principle applies to the process of finding and choosing a physician. Although the process of finding the right medical team requires a considerable investment in terms of both time and energy, the potential payoff can be well worth it. After all, what is more important than your health and well-being?

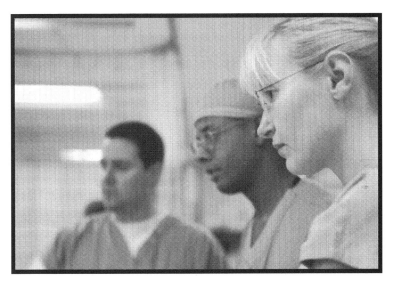

"Be the chief of staff of your medical team" -Melanie McDowell

PREPARING FOR A HOSPITAL STAY

Just as you take a "personal history" to your doctor visits, being prepared for emergency visit and hospital stays in a similar fashion is recommended. I have unfortunately been to the hospital too many times now. In the beginning, I did not go prepared. Nevertheless, through multiple visits, I have found a few things that allow me to get better treatment from the staff. A safe, smooth visit is exactly what you need when you are a chronic pain patient who is trying to heal or fight an illness.

For a better hospital stay, I now ask for a room in a quiet part of the hospital as sharp and sudden noises exacerbate my pain. Most hospital rooms now have their own thermostat so you can control your own temperature. If your room does not have its own, you can ask the nursing aide to assist with making you comfortable. If you are still not comfortable, you can also ask for warm blankets. When I am assigned a roommate I ask for my bed to be farthest from the door so that their visitors don't accidentally bump into me, and I can have less interruption with my resting. When possible, before their guests arrive, my husband or I inform them of my condition and how noise raises my pain levels. It is best to explain it to your roommate prior to his or her guest's arrival so that he or she may explain it to them for better cooperation. I have begun to bring in blankets and pillows from home. They are typically softer, and my quilts more comforting both in warmth and as a piece of home. With RSD, there is usually an increase in sweating, so just like at home, changing your sheets may need to be done more often. Some hospitals even offer a device to hold the blanket off your body areas w/ RSD. Most of the hospitals I have stayed in now offer an air mattress that can be used to adjust the bed to your preference. Comfort should be a big consideration so that you can heal faster.

It is almost unavoidable to not get poked with a needle as a patient in the hospital. They typically check blood at least once a day and use IV fluids to keep you hydrated. Medications are also administered with needles or through your IV. When they are drawing blood or putting in IV needles, ask for pediatric needles because any new trauma can cause RSD to spread to a new site. If a person takes my blood and I find them to be supportive and cooperative, I have asked that they be the one to check my blood every time. I even had a nurse who agreed to come in to take my blood specifically though she was off duty for one of the days I was in the hospital. It never hurts to ask for things that can make your stay more enjoyable and comfortable. When I had a pica line, I have asked them to take blood from it for less needle poking. While you are at it, have a nurse place a sign above your bed designating your affected limb(s). I had a nurse at the last hospital that also put a red bracelet on my unaffected limb and a red sticker on my chart for additional reminders for their staff. This served as a good reminder to the nurse and aides as they walked into the room. As they see multiple patients on your floor and as patients are coming and going often, you want to stay on top of your care. Employ the same "chief of staff" practices at the hospital that you do with your regular doctors. I request that the nurses only take blood and blood pressure from my left side, which is the least affected side. If you have both arms affected, ask the staff to use the thigh cuff. If you have bodywide RSD, specify the site you think will exacerbate the pain the least. A RSD friend suggested to me to have the hospital shave you and put in epidurals, catheter or other needed invasive items after anesthesia has begun. As the staff comes into the room, be sure to remind them to ask before they touch you so that you are prepared. If you are "out of it," have the person with you request this, or have a sign placed just outside the door so that they can see it before they come in. When you are going for X-rays or other tests that require transport, be sure to tell the transport staff what you need from them to best help you transfer to a wheelchair or bed, to help control pain from Hyperalgesia, and to watch bumps when going through doorways and onto the elevator. I always say, "My right side is affected, please do not touch me on that side, and if you have to run into something, please make it on the left." I also tell them, "If I fall, do not try to catch me, as it will hurt me worse. After I am on the ground, please pick me up using my left side only".

I also bring to the ER and hospital a list of medications. Sometimes I have had to have my own brought in. I think it is good to have my own supply there as well so I can control when I take them. Otherwise, have the nurse check with the hospital pharmacy to see if they carry all of your medications. I have found that nurses can't always be there at the appropriate time to administer medications or help with other needs due to an overload of patients. Therefore, if you have yours available, you can stay on schedule. I also have found that the hospital has charged me for taking my own medications, even when I brought them from home, although the cost will be less than having them providing you the medication. This can also save you from mix-ups in medications by their pharmacist. When you are on pain medication at the hospital, make sure to not wait until it is worn off before asking for more. Hospital staffs often times are taught to order your medications 30 minutes after you ask for them. Therefore, it could be 45 minutes or more before they actually arrive to your room from the time you ask for them. Keeping pain low is easier then lowering pain after it has skyrocketed again.

There are other considerations that can make your stay easier, more comfortable and insure proper treatment. Communication with your nurses, doctors and aides needs to stay calm, positive and corporative for the best possible treatment to be administrated. Try to have your nurse use warm alcohol or betadine wipes. They can warm them easily by rubbing them with their hands, running water on the outside of package before opening it or heating things in the microwave prior to application. For me, cold exacerbates the pain. After physical therapy exercises, the

PT used to tell me to wrap my shoulders with ice. It was very painful, and I would take it off as soon as I was told I could. Pain from ice was a new experience for me, as I had a knee injury in the past and used ice regularly to assist with swelling and gaining back function. It was very confusing as to why the ice bothered me so much with this new injury until I read in multiple sources that the ice can make RSD worse and possibly cause spreading.

Something I do at home is keep items on the bedside table for easy reach and use. In the hospital I use my tray table to serve the same purpose. I have it placed in a position so I do not bump it when resting but it is close enough to utilize it for my things. Also, if a nurse moves it to assist me or take blood pressure, I am sure to ask her to move it back into position when she is finished. Healthcare institutions that are accredited to assess and treat your pain have been mandated to treat pain as the fifth vital sign.[20] You have the right to be taken seriously, believed and demand pain control. If you feel that your needs are being overlooked or intentionally ignored, ask to speak with hospital administration as soon as possible. Remember to

---

[20] Joint Commission on Accreditation of Healthcare Organizations

be calm when making a statement or you may be the one that they do not take seriously.

In 2007, I was a patient at an Arizona Hospital for six days. On the third night, my IV infiltrated, and the nurses needed to put in a new one. The nurses on my floor were not able to do so because I have tiny veins that roll due to the circulation problems of RSD. Therefore, they called to have a pre-op nurse come up to do the insertion of the IV. When she arrived and began to prep me, I saw the IV needle and said, "I have RSD, and I need a pediatric needle. That looks like a large needle". She said, "This is a pediatric needle; it just looks big. Lay back and relax." She gave me a shot of Lidocaine and then inserted the needle. When she finished she proceeded to say, "I fooled you, haha, I used an adult needle, and see, it did not hurt." I said, "I have RSD. You told me it was a pediatric needle". Her response was, "I have people with RSV come into the pre-op all the time, and I give them this needle. Nothing will happen to you". I said, "I don't have RSV, I have RSD". She tried to blow it off with the sarcastic statement of, "Oh, Alphabet soup, I misspoke." I remarked, "If I get RSD in my left side because of you--" but she cut me off by, "You can't yell at me!" I finished, "It will be more than yelling..."

My husband and I were very upset at this point. The pre-op nurse just wanted to get out of the room. She picked up her supplies and walked out, but remained in the hall. Ken went to move my tray table back into place and noticed the used needle sitting on my table, covered with my blood. Ken and I were trying to snap a picture of it when the nurse saw this through the glass and came running back in. She said, "Opps, I did not finish the job," took the needle from Ken, and put it into the needle bin. When my regular nurse had come back, I told her what had happened and that I was very upset, and if the pre-op nurse causes my RSD to spread, how horrible it would be.

I was still very upset and in the morning, asked the new nurse on duty to call the hospital administration because I wanted to file a complaint. Later that day, I was visited by a charge nurse who took my statement. She said she would deal with it. When my regular night nurse came that night, she apologized again that the pre-op nurse used a "transfusion needle" on me and how it was not right. The next morning, I was transferred to a different floor.

193

My treatment was then phenomenal. I was worried that I would be treated poorly but was not. They took extra attention and care on my case. After I arrived home I filed a report with the state board of nursing. It took a year and five months but the nurse was brought before a board to defend herself. In my request, I was sure to say that I was not hoping for her to be fired, but instead to be required to attend a class on RSD and chronic pain so that she would understand what she had done to me and how serious it was. Fortunately for me, it did not cause any lasting problems. I have been in touch with other patients where this was the cause of their spread. It is very important to speak up before anyone touches you. Do so in a positive, educational manner, and they are usually receptive. If your challenges or pain are not taken seriously, or you are put into danger because of a healthcare professional, it is important to speak up; they will not learn unless you do.

KEY TO MEDICAL BILLING

Every time you see a medical provider and charges are run through your insurance or Medicare, you will receive a statement from the insurance company as well as the doctor's office. In a few pages, there is a sample insurance log, which is also known as an Explanation of Benefits (EOB). If you do not have insurance or Medicare, you can try to negotiate with the doctor for lower charges for underinsured or low-income patients.

The EOB statement contains: your providers name, date of service (DOS), procedure codes, billed charges, any negotiated discounts or savings, any non-covered charges and allowed charges, message codes, explanations, and total due including how much they paid and how much is the patient's responsibility.

- Be sure that the doctors billing office recognized any discounts or savings negotiated by your insurance. Finally, make sure that your amount due to the doctor does not exceed the amount stated on your EOB.

- Be sure to double-check the DOS, Procedure codes and billed charges.
- Be sure to match up the EOB and the doctors billing statement.

Learning how to spot errors and overcharges will save you time and money. Paying attention and catching the errors can radically cut your bill. The insurance logs are not always correct, and for that matter, doctor offices make billing mistakes as well. I have found on numerous occasions that I have saved thousands of dollars by doing my own comparison and finding the mistakes, instead of just paying the bill and not questioning the amount listed. Chances of finding an error are high. Medical Billing Advocates of America estimates that 8 out of 10 medical bills have errors.[21] No one should pay more than they truly owe for medical services, especially when it is not your mistake and you should be covered.

---

[21] Medical Billing Advocates of America, www.billadvocates.com

SAMPLE EXPLANATION OF BENEFITS

EXPLANATION OF BENEFITS (EOB)

THIS IS NOT A BILL

CONTRACT #	MEMBER NAME										
HPP504976	JOHN Q. SAMPLE			DATE 09/11/04							

CLAIM # / DATES OF SERVICE / PROVIDER NAME / PROCEDURE DESCRIPTION	PROVIDER CHARGE	AMOUNT DENIED	EX CODES	AMOUNT ALLOWED	APPLIED TO DEDUCTIBLE	COPAY OR PENALTY	COINSURANCE	OTHER INSURANCE	MEDICARE ALLOWED	MEDICARE PAID	AMOUNT PAID
0481890725720											
06/28/2004 - 06/28/2004											
JOHN Q. PROVIDER											
OFFICE VISIT FOR EXM, ESTABLISHED PATIENT 15 MINUTES	95.00	95.00	ZT	61.75	.00	.00	.00	.00	.00	.00	.00
ELECTROCARDIOGRAM ROUTINE ECG W AT LEAST 12 LEADS;W INTERPR	70.00	70.00	ZT	32.13	.00	.00	.00	.00	.00	.00	.00
	165.00	165.00		93.89	0.00	0.00	0.00	0.00	0.00	0.00	0.00

EXPLANATION OF CODE

EX CODE	
ZT	ENY-THE MEMBER IS INELIGIBLE AT THE TIME OF SERVICE-PATIENT LIABLE

									AMOUNT PAID
TOTAL AMOUNT PAYABLE TO PROVIDER(S) BY PLAN									0.00
TOTAL AMOUNT PAYABLE TO PROVIDER(S) BY MEDICARE									0.00
TOTAL AMOUNT PAYABLE TO PROVIDER(S) BY THIRD PARTY									0.00
TOTAL OF DEDUCTIBLE + COPAY + COINSURANCE WHICH IS PATIENT'S MINIMUM RESPONSIBILITY OWED TO PROVIDER									0.00

THIS IS NOT A BILL. An EOB provides information about how claims (bills for medical services) are processed. Keep this EOB for your records and, if applicable, use it to compare with actual provider bills.

Definitions to help understand this EOB.

Provider Charge: Amount provider (physician, hospital, etc.) bills for service.

Amount Denied: Amount _____ did not pay. May be due to our provider contract, your benefits coverage, lack of authorization or missing information.

EX Codes: Code assigned to the action taken on each service (e.g., a denial). Details provided in the Explanation of Code box above.

Amount Allowed: Amount eligible for payment consideration under our provider contract or payment guidelines. May be counted toward your deductible, if applicable.

Definitions (cont.)

Applied to Deductible: If your _____ coverage includes a deductible for this procedure, and your annual deductible has not yet been met, this is the portion of the bill you are responsible for paying to the provider.

Copay or Penalty: Amount you are responsible for paying to the provider. Penalties may occur when certain services are not authorized (e.g. surgery out of the network).

Coinsurance: Percentage of Amount Allowed that you are responsible for paying to the provider for this procedure, as determined by your coverage.

Other Insurance: Amount another insurance company is responsible for paying (e.g. worker's compensation or motor vehicle insurance).

Amount Paid: Amount _____ paid toward each service.

Refer to the Important Information section on reverse side for additional information.

On the preceding page, there is a sample EOB. You can see on this statement the important items to pay attention to:

1) Provider Name
2) Date Of Service
3) Procedure Description
4) Provider Charges
5) Amount Denied
6) Explanation Codes
7) Amount Allowed/Negotiated By Insurance
8) Amount Applied To Deductible
9) Co-Pay
10) Co-Insurance
11) Other/Secondary Insurance
12) Medicare Allowed/Medicare Paid
13) Amount Paid
14) Patient's Responsibility

Make sure to check each aspect of the EOB. The part to pay closest attention to is the Patient's Responsibility. Often times doctor's offices will send you a bill for anything not covered by the insurance. The problem is that your insurance company negotiated rates and discounts, and they keep track of what you actually owe. Comparing the EOB to the doctor's bill every time is a way to save thousands of dollars. I have done this myself and helped others do the same. On the next page there is a sample doctor's bill. Be sure that you understand both the EOB and doctor's bill, and you can also save thousands of dollars over time.

SAMPLE DOCTOR'S BILL

HOSPITAL ITEMIZED STATEMENT

PATIENT FINANCIAL SERVICES

	DATE OF BILL	DATE OF PREV. BILL	HOSP. NO	PAGE NO.
	07/12/06		050454	1

① **②** **③**

PATIENT NAME	ACCOUNT NUMBER	ADMISSION DATE	DISCHARGE DATE	DAYS
Patient Name	12345678	03/16/06		

ADDRESS SERVICE REQUESTED

Patient Name
Patient Address1
Patient Address2
City, State, Zip

C.D.E.	INSURANCE COMPANY NAME	GROUP #	POLICY NUMBER
		④	**⑤**
1	ABC Insurance		*******9999
	AMOUNT OF PAYMENT		$

○ FOR CHANGES IN PATIENT AND/OR INSURANCE INFORMATION, OR TO PAY BY CREDIT CARD, CHECK HERE AND COMPLETE THE BACK. PLEASE MAKE CHECKS PAYABLE TO   AND RETURN THIS PORTION WITH YOUR PAYMENT.

DATE OF SERVICE ⑥	QUANTITY ⑦	SERVICE CODE ⑧	DESCRIPTION OF HOSPITAL SERVICES ⑨	TOTAL CHARGES ⑩	AMOUNT BILLED TO INSURANCE 1 ⑪	AMOUNT BILLED TO INSURANCE 2 ⑫	PATIENT AMOUNT ⑬
DETAIL OF CURRENT CHARGES, PAYMENTS AND ADJUSTMENTS							
031606	1	4100101	COMP AUD THRSH EVAL & REC	200.00	200.00		
031606	1	4100251	TYMPANOMETRY	117.00	117.00		
031606	1	4100465	CONDITIONED PLAY AUDIOM	162.00	162.00		
BALANCE FORWARD				0.00			
SUMMARY OF CURRENT PAYMENTS/ADJUSTMENTS				0.00	0.00		
SUMMARY OF CURRENT CHARGES							
AUDIOLOGY				479.00	479.00		
TOTAL OF CURRENT CHARGES				479.00	479.00		

T O T A L S		
ACCOUNT NUMBER 12345678	(PLEASE REFER TO ACCOUNT NUMBER ON ALL INQUIRIES AND CORRESPONDENCE)	PAY THIS AMOUNT ⑮ 0.00

QUESTIONS? PLEASE CALL
MONDAY THROUGH FRIDAY, 9AM TO 3PM PST   TOTAL CHARGES = ⑯ 479.00

Additional patient billing may be necessary for any charges not posted when this bill was prepared, or if insurance carriers do not pay any part of the amounts billed to insurance. Based on income requirements, you may be eligible for a Government program, access to Charity Care, or Financial Assistance. For information please contact Patient Financial Services at

On the preceding page there is a sample doctor's bill. You can see on this statement the important items to pay attention to.

1) Account Number

2) Admission Date

3) Discharge Date

4) Insurance Company Name

5) Policy Number

6) Date of Service

7) Quantity

8) Service Code

9) Description of Services

10) Total Charges

11) Amount Billed to Insurance #1 (primary)

12) Amount billed to Insurance # 2 (secondary)

13) Patient Responsibility/ Amount Due

14) Summary of Current Charges

15) Pay This Amount

16) Total Charges

Again, use these to compare to the EOB. Also, if you have two insurance companies, make sure that the proper one is listed as the primary. If you have Medicare and an additional insurance company, there is an easy way to figure out which is the primary one. If the insurance is provided through a company with over 100 employees, then they are your primary and Medicare is secondary. I fall into this category. I have PPO insurance through my husband's employer and Medicare as my secondary. By comparing all three explanations (PPO, Medicare and doctor's bill), I have found additional mistakes and have saved even more money.

I have also negotiated a large bill with a hospital, so I know that it is possible to negotiate medical bills. You must be very organized and write a letter explaining your situation. Within a month of sending a letter to Catholic Charities, a caseworker was assigned to me and she worked with me to get this bill taken care of. I ended up owing nothing when all was said and done, and received back the money I had been able to send to the hospital. Although it was not much, it came in very handy towards paying my other medical bills.

The following is my letter to Catholic Charities, Community Services:

On September 26, 2002, I was in a minor auto accident. Since then, my life has dramatically changed. I was married at the time for 9.5 years, worked at a university as a head coach and ran a successful business. In the few seconds it took for the van to hit me in my car, it is amazing what damage it can do for a lifetime.

I lost my job, business, house, and most importantly my husband. My injuries have resulted in seven surgical procedures, five lung collapses, medical treatments in three different states, over $250,000 in medical bills, a huge change in my physical looks, physical abilities, and mental stability. I have been on welfare and am now on Permanent Social Security Disability. A place I never thought I would live through, but I have and I will. I understand that I am on a journey that has been pre-planned for me. Looking back on the last three years, I am in a better place now than I was with all of the "things" I had before the accident. I definitely know exactly what the people from New Orleans are going thru now and watching them on TV gave me a reflection on just how much I have overcome, *and I know that with God in my corner, everything will be okay.*

One of my experiences during this time was a full right lung collapse. This happened while I was at church. It was the first time I was able to leave my house/hospital in a month and my dad was here from VA taking care of me. He went out and found a church near my new home here in AZ. I was only out of the hospital for two days, but really wanted to go to church. The priest was asking the children some questions, and the kids were trying their best to answer. We all began to laugh at one particular answer. All of the sudden I could not breath and was in deep distress. Luckily, the church has a nurse who assisted me while waiting for the ambulance. At some point after that, my life flashed before me, and I realized that the most important thing in life is human connection and belief that God is in charge and everything will be okay no matter the outcome. I woke up after emergency surgery to put in a chest tube and my life has never been the same. I was able to let go of life's anxieties and complications that upset me so much before the accident. Although, I can't see God's plan, I know and believe that He knows more than me about what I need and what I can handle. I have finally been diagnosed with Thoracic Outlet Syndrome and Reflex Sympathetic Dystrophy. I am undergoing "treatment" about every five weeks to help with the extreme pain I live with daily.

I am now asking for help from Catholic Charities. I don't need "things." I need some assistance with my medical bills. There is one bill in particular. I was sent to Denver Colorado for my fourth surgery in May 04. This was a surgery done in a hurry to "fix" a problem from my first surgery (which was the cause of my five lung collapses). In my second surgery, my first rib was removed to assist with the symptoms of TOS and the bone that was left; it either began to grow or was not properly removed and was going in two directions. One was into a nerve bundle in my shoulder area and the other was into my lung. Wow, I thought that the second surgery was the last one and I was wrong.

I had ended up at Saint Luke's Hospital, Denver CO with a leading doctor for TOS. My doctors have been really understanding of my financial situation, some writing off what my insurance did not cover and others cutting my bills in half or more. My bill from St. Luke's Hospital was just over $34,000 and my insurance covered just over $19,000 *because the surgery was not pre-approved by the hospital. The hospital understood that I was in financial trouble and accepted payment of $26.23 on one account and $10 on the other, per month. I then received a call saying that I did not have to pay for now, because I showed my intent was to pay my debts as I never had missed a payment. I was going to be getting a settlement from the people responsible for my injuries and I could pay then. I have not received a settlement, and it could take years, if ever, if I do receive any compensation for my injuries at all. About three months after I stopped my payments my account was turned over to a collection agency, which is charging me interest. I then began to pay them the $36.23 each month. I began a new procedure about five months ago. They are experimental and are $4,800 per treatment most of which my insurance won't pay for since it is experimental. So I have to now make payments on these new treatments. However, these treatments are the first time I have received any relief from the pain since the accident, so they are worth it.*

I am on such a limited income and I am no longer able to pay the collection agency. As the interest is adding up, I see this debt growing and my payments meant *nothing. My mother who is a nurse in VA told me that sometimes, medical bills could be written off as charity by hospitals. I was wondering if Catholic Charities could assist me in requesting St. Luke's to take my case into consideration as a charity/hardship case. Please consider writing a letter to the hospital, or offer me any assistants and guidance that you may possess. The other doctors and facilities are taking my $10 payments each month and although it only means that I pay $120 a year to each of them they are willing to work with me. I pray to God and Jesus everyday to have his will be done and no longer worry about having a roof over my head or food to eat, because even though I don't have much, I have made it through to this point and know that God has my back, as he had never let me down. I look forward to your response and prayers.*

About a year later, I had an experience with an insurance company agent. Being a patient in a catastrophic case, I am conscious about making sure my medical bills are covered by insurance before receiving care, whenever possible. Most insurance companies define a catastrophic case as a patient with bills over $50,000. Making sure insurance will pay for my care allows me to better plan my budget so that I don't get in a large bill situation that I cannot fix, which would put a burden on me or my husband. Often times you may be pressured by insurance agents to get extra coverage or specific condition coverage.

If you already have health insurance, specific condition insurance is like duplicating coverage. Duplicate coverage is usually a waste of money because only one insurance will pick up the bill, and if you have two companies you're trying to use as primary companies, they may fight over who is responsible while in the meantime, you are responsible for the bills. Disease specific or accidental coverage is often times a waste. Your primary coverage usually covers more than the disease specific plan and will pay first, leaving you with a monthly premium for extra insurance that you did not need or get to use for the specific purpose of the coverage in the first place.

In September 2006, my husband and I felt we were misled by one of the local insurance agents when we were looking for medical insurance. I know mistakes happen, but health insurance is just such a major issue in my life that I had to let him know that I was very upset that he misled us and deceived us. In our initial conversation, I confirmed that the agent understood that I needed a major medical group health insurance plan that was PPO for small business owners or family, and I had to have a group plan that will cover my treatments. When the agent came to meet with us, we tried to ask questions. Each time he would change the subject or turn the page and tell us about something else. We made it clear that we were not in a hurry but were worried about obtaining a new group policy that would cover all of my needs. He basically "time-crunched" and diverted our attention, leaving us without getting all of our questions answered. We gave him the first month's premium plus the application fee, not realizing that he still never explained the policy he was putting us into. After he left, I began to read the pamphlet he had given us. We got suspicious when he called us just after leaving our house asking us when we wanted the coverage to begin. During this phone call, we started to ask some more questions that we thought he could just answer over the phone. One such question was should we increase our deductible to $3,000 from $1,000 so that we are not red-flagged by the company. This was one of the scare tactics he employed with us during our meeting, even to go as far as not wanting to list Medicare on the application, so that we could just get approved. He said, "Let's just get you through underwriting; because once you are through, they can't drop you". Had we done this and the insurance company found out, they would not have covered anything even if they had normally covered it. The other question was, "Is the deductible listed in the book correct"? If it meant what we thought, then every time I needed a procedure I would have to pay $3,000 vs. a onetime deductible per year with the other company I currently had, where my deductible was $100 per year (not co-insurance). At that point, he said he was turning around and coming back so he could get a new check for the higher deductible. We are glad that he did come back, because it gave me more time to think. When he arrived Ken was writing the check for the new amount as I began asking more questions. We had never discussed ambulance coverage; I did not know what a co-insurance maximum meant; what percentage of the bill the insurance company pays after I pay the initial $3000; and which additional plan options were listed for us. I also noticed that there were other rider options listed in the pamphlet that were not discussed as additional possible needs. He again did not answer my questions. His response this time was, "We can add that stuff later. We just need to get you approved first, and that is our main goal." He then reminded me of our earlier conversation where he told me to not express to the insurance agent who calls, all of my medical issues, at which time I said I want to be totally open because having the right coverage was so important to me. He then told me not to give any further information to the agent than what is asked of me, or that I would not be approved for any coverage.

As an RSD patient, correct coverage is very important. That agent either did not know the product he was selling, or he was deceiving and misleading many customers. Leaving us to believe the coverage he signed us up for will cover my doctor and hospital visits of a more acute nature was very deceptive. We thought he was listening to us, helping us come up with a policy that would meet our needs.

The point of my story is that just because you have insurance does not guarantee that you will be covered for the services you need. Nowadays, businesses are cutting back on the coverage they purchase for their employees. Make sure you check your policies for over- and under-coverage and for what you are able to cover with your insurance. Spending some time to look over your policy in advance can save you time and money in the long run.

TIPS

- Don't buy disease specific or accident insurance.
- Don't duplicate coverage.
- Get pre-approval for services such as procedures/surgeries and durable medical equipment.
- Negotiate with hospitals and other providers.
- Only use providers who accept your medical plan.
- Pay premiums on time.
- Seek financial resources you can turn to for help.

When you have a catastrophic injury or illness, it is important to learn how to negotiate effectively with your healthcare provider for lower costs of care, especially when you do not have medical insurance or are a cash patient.

Negotiating Your Bill:

- Ask about the cheaper alternatives.
- Pay ahead of time, cash if possible.
- Shop around.
- Use your doctor as your advocate; don't be afraid to ask for a reduction in your bill.
- Work out a payment plan.

Before you go in for care, compare prices for the treatment from multiple doctors in your area. This may not be possible if it is an emergency situation. It is beneficial to have a realistic cost in mind when starting to negotiate pricing. Note that charges are incurred for every area of service. Service areas include doctors (your surgeon, anesthesiologist, surgical assistants and any other doctor your surgeon asks to be in on the surgery), nurses, facility, medications, supplies and even the food they provide in a hospital room. Everything you receive is chargeable including bedding, having your room cleaned, medication (each pill is billed separately), and IV bags. You would be surprised at the details they keep on you, which are then coded and given to the billing department. Often times, you can get the same procedure at a surgical center or doctor's office surgical suite for a fraction of the cost. Be sure to check all avenues available for your procedure. Also remember, if you have insurance, check to see if the doctor you are using AND the facilities are both covered by your insurance. I have found out after a procedure that my doctor's billing was covered, but the hospital was not an approved hospital under my plan. This can be very costly.

When going outside of your insurer's network, doctor's fees can be very expensive. Most doctors leave their billing up to an assigned staff person. The doctor is there to treat the patients and, although they will probably make the final decision on pricing for their services, the billing staff will be whom you negotiate with. Make sure to be courteous and speak slowly while fully explaining your situation. If you see this doctor often, you don't want the staff to have a negative view of you, which will impact your relationship with the doctor. If after working with the billing office your request is denied, then it would be okay to bring it up to the doctor directly. Again, use tact and professionalism. Be unassuming and appreciative even if they offer you less than what you were asking. You can

214

always tell them, "I will think about it and let you know if I can work that into my budget." They may also be willing to make payment plans. Doctors like it when a patient is upfront about finances. Healthcare is a service industry. Just as you would negotiate the rate you pay your plumber for fixing your pipes, it is okay to make a similar request to the healthcare provider.

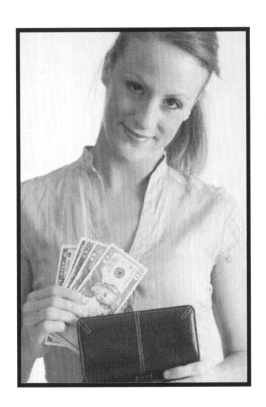

Of course, paying in cash will be a helpful way to negotiate. If you have cash in hand and say you can pay a certain amount right away, then they are more likely to make a deal than if you have to ask for a discount and then spread it out over time. If you do take a payment plan option, be sure that you know what kind of interest will be applied to the balance, if any. When you are paying with a credit card, it costs the doctors money for processing, and therefore cash over cards would probably lead to a lower discount offered.

I would bet most doctors don't know the exact cost of the tests, procedures or prescriptions they are asking you to fill. I have had situations where I found that a doctor was undercharging and another doctor who was priced triple what other doctors in the area were charging. I mentioned it to both of them, and they seemed receptive, especially the doctor who had the lower costs. Doing your own research can also help keep your bills down. You may come across another choice that is just as good but half the price. The doctor may also be able to suggest less expensive alternatives. Be sure you know if there are any limitations or drawbacks to the lower alternative.

RECAP

- As soon as you know your procedure has been scheduled, call the billing office to discuss prepayment for a self-pay surgery, pricing and payment plans.
- Ask for a discount rate on any additional fees associated with an overnight stay, if that becomes necessary.
- Ask your doctor if there are any alternatives available.
- Find out if there is a set discount if you pay in full prior to surgery.
- Write down the exact amount and the name of the person you talked to and ask them to make sure it is put on your record.
- You can save more if you befriend the doctor and his staff.

PATIENT RIGHTS

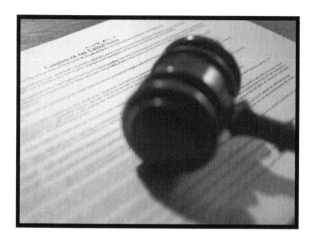

Often times I run into patients who have been treated poorly or perceive they have been treated poorly. I have included this section on the Patient's Bill of Rights so you know what to expect from your doctor. Doctors often times see a large number of patients each day. If you feel that some doctors are not listening to you, not understanding you, or being rude, try talking to them about it. Often times they are just running behind schedule, have something personal in their life going on, or even are upset that they can't help you more. Your reaction to what you perceive can play a part in the care you receive.

The more respect and consideration you can give the healthcare staff the more compassionate that they can be for your situation. Considerate and respectful care means that the healthcare professional is understanding, caring, and thoughtful. They show these attributes by being polite, considerate and courteous. You should also show them respect even when you're feeling bad or not heard.

You have a right to your records. I order my medical records from my providers after each visit. In some states, they are able to charge you for such copies. In Arizona, where I live, the law is if you're using them for future care, they cannot charge you. Check with your state for the law on this practice. I keep all of my records so that I can bring the ones needed to new doctors and can also refer back to them to double check a medication for past reactions and usefulness.

You should also check your records for mistakes. Healthcare professionals, like all humans, also don't always take perfect notes or a person transcribing their notes into your file can make a mistake. It states that it is important to do your own research about recommended treatments, and you can refuse care in most cases. Your healthcare provider needs to inform you of the risks you are taking by not following the recommendation they have made. If you're not comfortable, speak up prior to service.

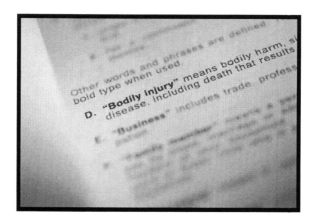

Records are confidential unless there is a risk to you or others or in a court case where they are used as admissible evidence. There is more in your records than medical information. Doctors write in their records more than just physical assessments. They write down your demeanor, if you were dressed appropriately, if your hair is brushed, if you were upset, anxious or combative, and so on. It is in their opinion and discretion as to how they perceive you. In 1996, the United States Department of Health and Human Services (U.S. - D.H.H.S.) issued a

220

privacy rule, which was finalized by the Secretary of Health and Human Services in 2000. The U.S. - D.H.H.S. is the official central governmental hub for all Healthcare Insurance Portability and Accountability Act (HIPAA) issues including rules, standards and implementation guides. Keeping HIPAA privacy laws enforced can assist you in receiving proper care and from letting outsiders like your employer or others know your personal health.[22]

The American Academy of Pain Management has also developed a Patient Bill of Rights. "It is an expectation that compliance with the Patient's Bill of Rights can contribute to an effective program for the patient. All pain management activities are to be provided with an overriding concern for the patient, and above all, with the recognition of the patient's dignity as a human being."[23]

As a patient, I expect to receive attention and respect from my healthcare providers. I have the right to considerate care and to expect that they will follow through. If the provider does not, then I find a new one,

---

[22] Healthcare Insurance Portability and Accountability Act, .U.S. Department of Health & Human Services See 45 CFR 164 AKA Code of Federal Regulation 45, 164

[23] American Academy Of Pain Management Patient's Bill Of Rights, aapainmanage.org

which I have had to do in the past. I have had a doctor say, "I know what you're trying to do, and you will not get away with it." He did not perform any tests on me, but when records were ordered, it turned out that there were results from a test that I did not undergo. When either provider or patient shows disrespect, proper treatment will be hard to accomplish. When communicating with my providers, I hope that they will give me complete and current information, but do not always expect it. I have learned that it is also important to research information on your own.

Your doctor should be expressing his final diagnosis, proposed treatment and expected prognosis in layman's terms so it is easy to understand. In some cases, I have had doctors share the information with my husband because they could see that I was not able to concentrate due to the pain, and it was important to have the information so that we could better prepare for what was to come. After this information is shared with my husband or me, we do our own research. In the beginning, I did what every doctor told me to do whether it was something I wanted to do or not. I learned through trial and error that I have the right to refuse any medical treatment. I listen to the doctor about medical consequences for my decision but no longer expect the doctor to make any final decisions for me.

Before a procedure, I want to know why the expected procedure would be an option, what are the benefits and drawbacks, if there is anything else available that could give me similar benefits with fewer risks, if my doctor will be bringing in any assistance for the procedure, and how many times the doctor has performed this procedure on other patients. I also want to know how long the recovery is and what is entailed in the recovery. Will it be a few days or will it be months of physical therapy?

I like to know if the procedure is experimental. For instance, the Radiofrequency Ablation I undergo is considered experimental by insurance for RSD. Most treatments for RSD are experimental because there is not one thing that "cures" it and insurance company caseworkers are not always on top of what specific procedures are helpful for a patient. I have had to write letters and have my doctors write letters to explain why a particular procedure or medical intervention is appropriate for me and fight to get coverage. I have been in a situation where a doctor has not done many of the procedures, or wants to perform research or a biopsy to share the informational aspects with others. I have signed papers to release some of my records for this purpose and have also had students attend some of my surgeries to observe what my surgeon was doing so that they could use the experience as a learning tool.

If you are in a position to injure yourself or others, then there are some laws that govern the doctor to perform medical intervention without consent, but in most situations it is up to you or your medical proxy to make the decision. I noticed that in my records when I underwent a procedure or surgery, the doctor would write, "the patient has elected to have the surgery performed after I explained the risks and benefits to her." However, from my perspective, the doctor was telling me that I had to have the procedure, and I did not have a choice. In some of the cases, I would not have had the procedure had I known my rights. I now know that I have the right to receive all information the doctor has on the medical plan being offered and that I also can have time to think about what I want to do, thus, allowing for my own research and decision-making.

Finally, I expect to have my doctors communicate with each other about my treatment plan.   It can help facilitate greater care, less medication mix-ups and fewer complications. When everyone works together as a team with me leading it, I know I am getting the best care possible. Prompt and proper pain management is a basic healthcare right and you, as a patient, should not settle for anything less.

GOING TO THE DENTIST

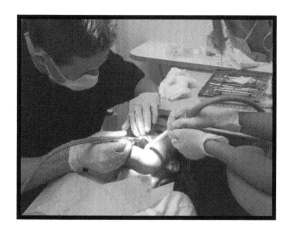

Going to the dentist can be frightening for anyone. With RSD you should pay extra attention when choosing your dentist. It is important that the dentist you choose knows about RSD. Considerations your dentist needs to know before treating you, or even cleaning your teeth, include: your diagnosis as a RSD patient, medications you are taking, any allergies, and your vulnerability to infection as your immune system is compromised because you live with chronic pain.

Be sure to report vitamins, supplements, over-the-counter drugs, and prescription medications to your dentist.

Your dentist can help you understand any potential dental health side effects that may occur as a result of taking medications or combinations of medications. Being prepared can help you avoid the downfalls of medication on your teeth. For instance, Neurotin is known to yellow the teeth. Find out from your dentist what you can do to help prevent these and other downfalls. Other downfalls include dry mouth syndrome, periodontal disease and tooth decay.

Oral care starts with good practices at home. If brushing hurts, try closing your eyes and concentrating on breathing or your plans for the day. Problems when dealing with chronic pain can also come into play when a patient is frequently vomiting, has poor brushing habits and a lack of financial stability. Poor brushing can come from a loss of range of motion, a patient not feeling good enough to brush, or because it causes increased pain. Finding ways to brush properly and more often will help you keep your teeth longer. I suggest the use of an electric toothbrush. You can hold it to each tooth without having to move your arm back in forth. Using fluoride toothpaste and mouthwash can also help. A side effect of medication can be vomiting, and even high pain levels can cause nausea and vomiting. According to the Better Health Channel,[24] brushing after vomiting can break down the enamel on your teeth faster as well as cause scratches. After vomiting try rinsing with drinking water followed up by a fluoride rinse or mouthwash. My dentist, Dr. Huang, was able to provide me with pure fluoride with a pump and small cap. I take a small amount of fluoride mixed with water and swish it for 2 minutes after an unpleasant vomiting experience. You can also take a bit of toothpaste and use your finger to smear it on your teeth and gums, then rinse. Dr. Haung, suggests waiting to brush at least an hour after vomiting. This helps save your enamel from early decay and helps prevent oral infections.

As far as financial issues, most dentists will allow you to pay with monthly payments and give you a cash discount. One complaint I hear from disabled patients is that Medicare does not offer dental coverage. Oral health is so important, but coverage may be hard to get. It is expensive, but finding a way to have your teeth cleaned at least twice a year can really help prevent other more expensive problems from occurring.

---

[24] Better Health Channel Health and medical information for consumers, quality assured by the Victorian government (Australia).

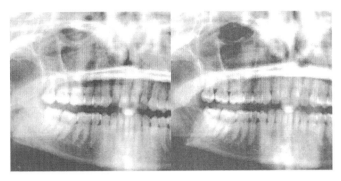

Barby's facial x-ray from the dentist 2004 and 2006.
Note the dystrophy and thinning bone above the top jaw.

Keep in mind that any invasive procedure, including dental work, can cause RSD to worsen. It is important to control your pain before, during and after the procedure. While at the dentist, you can ask for numbing solutions such as Lidocaine or sedation, even for teeth cleanings. Keeping oral pain to a minimum or even non-existent will help keep your stress and chronic pain at a manageable level. Nowadays, there are many techniques that a dentist can use so that you feel no pain or minimal discomfort. If you begin to feel pain while the dentist is still working on your teeth, it would be good to arrange a signal ahead of time, like raising a hand or finger to let the dentist know you are feeling pain. Take advantage of the free toothbrush and floss many dentists will provide to you after your

229

cleaning. If they don't give you a soft bristled toothbrush, ask if they have any available.

I find that I cannot keep my mouth open for long periods of time. Don't be afraid to let the dentist know if you need "close your mouth breaks". The staff can work on other patients and come back to you, as you are able to tolerate additional dental work or cleaning. Your teeth are an important part of your overall health.

There are ways to control the pain of dentistry for RSD patients through medications and other tools coming down the pipeline. Dentists are working hard to create tools for all patients to receive better oral care treatment with less pain. "They're working on a non-thermal plasma brush that uses a low-temperature chemical reaction to disinfect and prepare cavities for filling." In typical (and often painful) cavity repairs, the dentist drills away the affected area and then makes a filling to restore the tooth's shape. The brush will operate without the heat and vibrations that cause the pain and discomfort associated with the current procedure.[25] As an RSD patient, be sure to speak up about your

---

[25] Pain-Free Dentistry, September 13, 2007, Scout News, LLC. Health Day News

condition before the dentist begins. They are typically good at accommodating you as a pain patient.

RECAP

- Ask for "close your mouth breaks" if needed.
- Brushing after vomiting can break down the enamel.
- Have your teeth cleaned at least twice a year.
- It is important for your dentist to know about RSD.
- Oral care starts at home.
- Poor brushing can come from a loss of range of motion or just not feeling good enough to brush or brushing causing increased pain.
- Use an electric toothbrush as a way to achieve proper brushing.
- Your dentist needs to know that you are an RSD patient, all medications you are taking, any allergies, and that your vulnerability to infections.

SOCIAL SECURITY DISABILITY

Many RSD patients become disabled and unable to work a job to support themselves, their family and their new medical bills. If you need to file for Social Security Disability (SSD) or Social Security Income (SSI), there is a process. I completed this process without a lawyer, but know others who chose to use one. If you are truly disabled, the best situation would be to find quick access to benefits and medical care. It does not always work that smoothly. When filing, fill out every piece of information requested. Gathering your own records and sending them with your application speeds up the process. The SSD offices will request these records, and it takes time for them to process the request, send them to the doctors, get them back and process the receipt of them. Sending them in from the start cuts a lot of the time that these processes would take. Some things can help your chance of winning the first time you apply for disability. Using an attorney will cause you to lose some of the benefits you would receive because they take their pay for helping you from the benefits.

When you are ready to apply, fill out the forms and bring a copy to your doctor(s). Find out if they will support you. If they will, ask them for a statement to help support your case. Make sure they include why you are disabled and unable to work. Submitting these with your application will help the process along. If the SSD office asks you for more information or records, comply in a timely manner. Cooperate fully with the SSD caseworker on your case by having a helpful, positive attitude, responding promptly to letters and notices, and going to requested medical exams as soon as possible. I was asked to do an exam prior to receiving my benefits.

Keep in touch with your caseworker. They have many cases in their load, so staying at the top of the file will help your process speed up. Call for updates. When you call, record the conversation or take notes as to whom you spoke to, what their title is, what department they are in, the date, time and what their answer to your questions were. Also, ask them when they think this part of the process will be completed. Tell them you will call back to check if you do not hear anything by then. It is good to call for updates on an initial claim, reconsideration or receipt of additionally requested information. Be sure to call the department that is processing your paperwork at that time. The case moves through multiple stages while being evaluated. Keep up-to-date on deadlines, and if you think you may miss a deadline, call and let them know. Also, ask if you can fax or email the paperwork in for quicker processing. By maintaining a good working relationship with the caseworkers (claim representatives and the case examiners), they are more willing to help you, and you will find the process easier and manageable without assistance from an attorney. If you feel that you are being over looked or unfairly evaluated, consider writing to your senator for assistance. If your case is denied, find out why and correct the information before reapplying. It is always good to contest a decision and not give up. Persistence is part of the process in receiving the benefits you deserve.

SECTION FOUR

TIPS & TRICKS FOR COPING WITH RSD

PAIN IN PERSPECTIVE TO LIFE

Taking each challenge one step at a time can help you gain perspective on your future: a focus on mental and physical health, trends in the healthcare industry, research projects available and personal injury liability. There are multiple aspects to pain management to be learned and considered. Putting life into perspective can help us deal with the behavioral changes, social isolation and our spiritual concerns.

Understanding that pain causes depression, not the other way around, can be a good place to start. Realize that you have control over your actions, and feeling bad is not a proper excuse for treating others poorly. Doing so can lead to social isolation. You may not feel like having others around is helpful, or it may make you self-conscious about losing the ability to do daily activities of life. Creating a support network and staying socially involved can increase your quality of life as an RSD'er as well as increase the human connection, which we all need. Once again, I need to emphasize proper communication for better treatment, attitude, and comfort. Working with your social network, finding out about future trends and what your doctor has recently learned can help you keep the pain perspective.

Have hope that a cure will develop. If a new procedure becomes available, you will be prepared and have the support of those around you. When you hear of positive news like a new procedure, ask your doctor about them and if they will perform the procedure. Find out if it is just another gimmick or if there is real science behind it. Be sure to do your own research and be comfortable with your choices. With RSD, more than ever you have to be your own advocate and motivate others to advocate for you. If you were injured through someone else's negligence, find out the legal consequences and if any action can be taken. Speak with a personal injury attorney to find out if you have a case. If you do, he can instruct you on how to arrange payments for medical treatments and how the lawyer will be paid. Question if the defendant is responsible for your bills now or if you have to find a way to cover your medical bills and be paid back when and if you win your case. Also, it is important to know what happens if you don't win your case. Ask if you will have to pay back charges your lawyer paid to prepare the case, if you have to pay liens if you lose your case. Liens are holds or rights to property or monetary gain on property. Many doctors' offices will put liens on your case. This means that they get paid before you receive any winnings or awards.

Becoming prepared for these new life changes will keep the perspective to your new life on a positive track. Use your community resources such as food banks, church supports and non-profit support to get the help you need. Help is there; you just have to be willing to take it and put in as much as you can to keep your life on track. Because chronic pain and bad health in general weakens the immune system, your ability to heal and fight diseases is also compromised. I very often can catch someone's cold by being near them through physical contact such as hugs or sharing candy out of the same dish as a child who has dirty hands. Often as a pain patient I do not want others to touch me, both for my health and because, unless they really know me, they don't know where it hurts and can make me worse really quick. So I usually ask people not to touch me without asking. Be prepared to face the pain and have a plan.

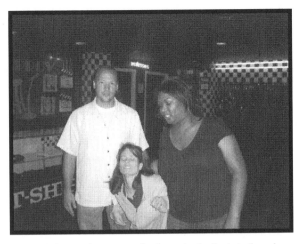

After being touch unexpectedly, I react instinctively to the pain

Lifestyle Changes

- As a coping tool, I ask myself what can I do to get myself through this challenge

- Financial aspects start with not being able to buy what I want, when I want to, and sometimes I can't even buy what I need.

- I have to make conscious decisions to work through the life changes chronic pain brings on a daily basis.

- Legal aspects that can last for years, with no guaranteed outcome, take a toll on you with stress and preparations.

- Loss of many childhood friends because they just did not understand what I was going through.

239

- My pain can interfere with important and enjoyable parts of life, which leads to a poor quality of life and can cause: clouded thinking, physical limitations, job problems, people problems, unpleasant moods, and spiritual distress. This reduces the quality of life for family, my friends and me.

- Pain Affects Your Mind, Body & Spirit!

Activity Level

- Pain wears me out and limits my activity level. I have to prepare before events and outings by allowing time to rest before and after, making it difficult to be active for two or more days in a row.

- Try to do what you can and find your limitations and boundaries. I have been assisted with this through my use of note taking and watching a pattern form from the activities I have tried to accomplish.

- Your ability to work and play decreases. In turn, our physical relationships suffer on every level (Family, Friends and Sexual).

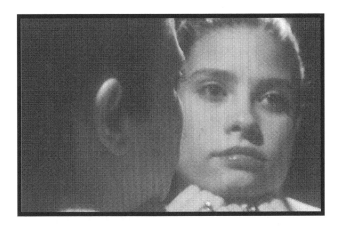

Physical Health

- I am weaker physically, and I find it easier to get sick, as the constant chronic pain has also affected my immune system.

- I have changed my life, as I now need help opening items and lifting even light objects. I have changed to paper plates and cups to reduce dropping them, drinking out of straws, and having my husband prepare meals before leaving the house so I am able to eat when he is not home to assist me.

- Pain affects coordination, balance and physical strength. I have fallen many times since getting RSD. I am not exactly sure as to why, but have found this to be a common problem with other RSD patients as well. Dizziness plays a part in the falls, but I also have trouble with vision, and medications, probably, have some role as well.

Overall Well-being

- Ability to sleep and rest
- As my pain increases, my nausea and vomiting also increase, a common side effect of chronic pain and some medications, which can lead to poor eating.
- For me, stress intensifies the pain and my ability to relax becomes diminished.
- I get into a bad pain cycle and can't sleep for days at a time. Without a good sleep cycle, you cannot function properly for long. When sleep is interrupted by chronic pain, it leads to insomnia, poor decision-making and bad moods. In turn, our emotional relationships suffer, and the pattern continually gets worse as the sleep cycle is compromised.
- My overall sense of well-being seems to be compromised.

HELPFUL TIPS TO USE EVERYDAY

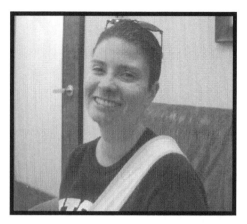

Barby waiting to be seen by a doctor, 2004

In order to remain as independent as possible and to minimize the disruption of daily life, individuals with RSD will need to consider changes to their daily routine and also in their surroundings. For example, for the person with lower extremity RSD, getting around can cause a significant challenge since doing normal activities can be quite painful. Activities such as walking, taking the stairs, squatting, sitting for long periods, and getting in and out of vehicles become a challenge. Every patient and their family should assess the surroundings, perhaps with the help of professionals, and prioritize the modifications needed. This

243

can help the patient maintain their independence and function. Some of the lifestyle modifications that patients with RSD may wish to consider include:

- Clothing
  - Flat shoes instead of heels for patients with lower extremity RSD
  - Slip-on shoes
  - Velcro or zipper closures for shirts or sweaters
  - Velcro or zippers for shoes instead of shoelaces
- Bathroom
  - Elevated toilet seat
  - Grab bars in the bathtub, shower, and next to the toilet
  - Long-handle comb or brush so the patient does not have to raise his or her arm high
  - Tub or shower bench
- Bedroom
  - Blanket support frame so that blankets or sheets do not rest directly on the feet of a patient
  - Nightlights in the bedroom and any other rooms where the patient may walk if they awaken during the night

- Automobile
  - Car doors that are easy to open and close
  - Handicapped parking stickers
  - Modified controls to facilitate driving
  - Seat positions that are easy to manipulate
- Kitchen
  - Easy grab handles for cabinets
  - Large knobs on appliances requiring manipulation (e.g., stove, dishwasher, washing machine)
  - Lightweight appliances (e.g., vacuum cleaner)
  - Lightweight dishes and pots
  - Lightweight flatware with long handles
  - Long handled cleaning appliances, (e.g., brooms, dustpans, sponges)
  - Long-handled "grabbers" for removing items on high shelves or picking up items from the floor
  - Sliding shelves or turntables on kitchen shelves so the patient does not have to reach into cabinets to access items at the back of a shelf

- Miscellaneous
  - A note from your doctor recommending special accommodations, such as an aisle seat in airplanes
  - Electric wheelchair to avoid upper body strain or injury
  - Medical support professionals or accountants to budget medications, special appliances, home-nursing care, and other medical-related supplies and expenses
  - Nursing or home health care
  - Use of wheelchairs in airports, train stations, or malls
  - Voice activated lights, appliances, or computer
  - Wheelchair-access modifications at home

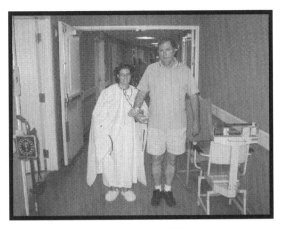

Barby in hospital, 2005

Undoubtedly, there has been progress made in recent years by healthcare professionals and patients towards understanding and properly managing pain. Unfortunately, pain still poses a problem for patients who are under-diagnosed, over-diagnosed or misdiagnosed. Controlling the pain you are in is essential to quality of life. Knowing the characteristics of pain and why it is happening give you an advantage in dealing and controlling aspects of pain. Taking control of your life and being responsible for yourself will assist you in lowering your pain.

HOW TO COMPLETE A JOURNAL

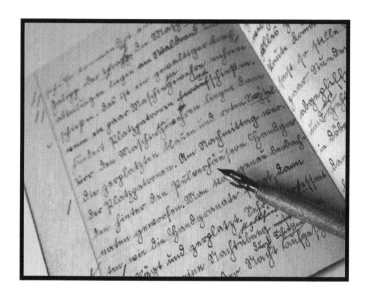

Understanding why your body is reacting as it does and the roles of the brain and the nervous system are the best ways to help yourself. Dealing with everyday stresses takes tools that most of us have not practiced in the past but quickly have to adapt to in order to manage our new reality. Knowing your treatment options, causes of your pain, how it can be properly diagnosed and long-term care needed, will give you support as well as the ability to help yourself. Keeping track of how you are doing with activities of daily living, symptoms you are experiencing after the start of RSD as well as when your healthcare professionals are treating you is a good idea. Below are some excerpts from my records, to give you an idea of where to start.

Symptoms from Car accident

October 2002

- Blackouts
- Can't work to full duties
- Disorganized thought w/ headaches, trouble focusing
- Ear pain R/L (off and on)
- Facial numbness (off and on)
- General sleep problems due to pain and discomfort, taking sleeping pills
- Headaches (off and on)
- Husband drives me around due to blackouts
- Husband has to help wash my hair
- Inability to turn head quickly
- Jaw pain
- Neck/back pain daily
- Pain/numbness when raise R arm in arm and fingers

249

- Problems looking down to read and write
- Shoulder pain on L
- Shoulder pain on R, going into arm
- Vision/Hearing Affected during blackouts

November 2002

- Same as last month
- Missed work
- Numbness in hands/ fingers (off and on)
- Passed out/ hit head, lead to hospital visit

December 2002

- Same as last month

On a daily level when figuring out my activity limitations, I kept track of pain levels, medications, and doctor visits in the morning and evening each day.

Date	PAL Morning	PAL Night	Other
28-Jan	4	6	PT w/ED, 400 mg. IB, Started new exercises
29-Jan	3	3	400 mg. IB
30-Jan	2	9	PT w/ED, Pain all the way to fingers after PT, headache (jaw, ear, behind eye), 400 mg. IB, Tape on back
31-Jan	4	6	400 mg. IB, Tape on back
1-Feb	4	6	400 mg ib, tape on back
2-Feb	6	8	400 mg ib, took tape off
3-Feb	7	9	Dr. French, New tape, trouble sleeping, 400 mg ib, took sleep pill still had trouble sleeping, started me on seizure meds.
4-Feb	6	6	No hand numbness the whole day, New tape, trouble sleeping, 400 mg ib, took sleep pill still had trouble sleeping
5-Feb	4	6	Tape makes difference, 3 separate pains (Neck, R arm, upper left arm), 400 mg ib
6-Feb	5	7	Pt w/ED, 400 mg ib, New tape

PREPARING TO TRAVEL

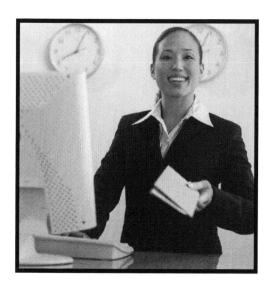

In traveling nowadays, there are overcrowded terminals, flight delays, and security with which we have to contend. There are ways to make traveling easier and less stressful for chronic pain patients. My first suggestion is to pack your medications in a carry-on bag. If your luggage gets lost, you won't have to worry about where or how to get your medications. As travel terminals are hectic and people are at a frantic pace, arriving early so you can go at a slower, more relaxed pace will make the hassles of dealing with disabilities manageable when traveling. Your

252

goal is to make it to your destination on time, in a low pain level and in a good mood. When you decide to make a trip, it is best to plan ahead. I use the Internet to get destination information. I check out the floor plans of the airports I am coming and going from, and what types of foods are available in the terminals. I also request handicapped services from the airline, bus depot, car rental company, and hotel all ahead of time.

My mother is on oxygen and has had a few troubles traveling because of it. If you are on oxygen, let the airline know 30 days prior to travel or as soon as you know that you will be flying. In-flight oxygen needs to be prearranged, and there is typically a charge. Then call 24-48 hours prior to your flight to confirm the oxygen arrangements. At the airport, if traveling alone, bring tip money. I try to bring one-dollar bills and tip a dollar for each bag that I am assisted with, both when I am departing and at my destination. I also pay the person pushing my wheelchair one to two dollars for their assistance. I also have a scooter, so I do not always have to pay for the wheelchair assistance. It is not mandatory to pay for help; however, the person pushing you often works for tips only or tips with a low wage. Be sure to let them know if you want to make any stops to use the restroom or purchase food while they are assisting you. When they bring you to your gate, ask to be "parked" at the door or the start of the line. Make sure that the airline person sees you. If you sit off to the side, they may miss you, and you will not be able to take advantage of pre-boarding. If you need extra time and assistance, you may have a problem. Typically, the flight attendant or ground crew comes over to me and moves me up in the plane if I have a seat towards the back, and they ask me if I need any assistance walking, or if I need an aisle chair to get to my seat. I do not tip the attendant who brings me down the jet way. When I pre-board, once on the plane, if I need to take medication or I am nauseated, I ask for a small glass of water. I also board with the first group, when they call for people who need assistance. If they do give you a small glass of water, they must take it back before the plane takes off; make sure you drink what you need when they give it to you.

Let them know while in flight if you need assistance in using the restroom or need blankets and pillows for comfort. When you arrive at your destination, stay in your seat until your wheelchair assistance has arrived. They typically ask you to wait until the other passengers unload so that you do not hold them up or so that they do not bump against you and cause you further injury. At baggage claim, if you are alone, ask the assistant to get your luggage and to bring you outside to meet your party. Once you are in a place you do not need assistance, give them their tip and thank them, so they may go help other travelers needing assistance.

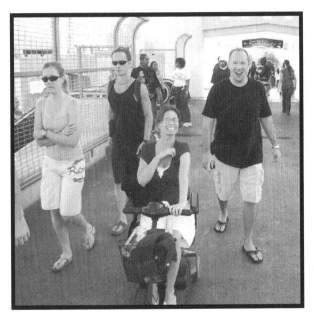

Barby and her husband on their honeymoon, Nov. 2007

FINAL THOUGHTS

You are your own advocate and must be in charge of your care. The responsibility of your well-being starts with you and then incorporates your caretaker and professionals. Communicating effectively is the key to better treatment from family, friends and healthcare providers. Start by being organized and structured in your daily activities. This can save you time and stress in your everyday life, get your quality time with your healthcare providers, and save you money. It will take some thought and preparation, and then you just need to maintain the system you create.

There are many options available to patients. Be sure to do your own research, and make sure your information is current. Use resources such as doctors, the Internet, other patients, caretakers, journal articles and books. I wish each of you the best life possible, the best healthcare possible and the best health possible. Remember, you are not alone in this circumstance, and you can reach out to other patients, as we need human connection now more than ever.

APPENDIX

ACKNOWLEDGEMENTS

I would like to acknowledge those who have helped me through this life-changing ordeal of RSD in significant ways. First and foremost, the Holy Trinity, God our Father, Jesus his son and the Holy Spirit for his strength and guidance when I am weak; for taking away my anxiety and allowing me to create the tools to cope with RSD. My faith has kept me on a strong spiritual path. Without the knowledge that I am saved and that everything will be ok and I just have to keep LIVING, I would have had many times that I could have given up.

My husband Ken, who has stood by me before we were even dating and has helped me every step of the way on a daily basis. He has been a dream and the most supportive of all the caretakers I know. Other patients and caretakers look up to him as much as I do, and he is great beyond words.

My father Jim who has been there for me while I was growing up as well as through my RSD ordeal. He traveled to me for most of my surgeries and my lawsuit and has started the Power of Pain Foundation, actively spreading awareness and education of RSD. My husband and I have been able to turn to him for moral support and advice, and he has always been there for me. He helped me create the Wisdom of Ingle book as a project to document our family history and to offer a light-hearted read to readers. This project kept me busy for many years and gave me a project when I needed to get my mind off of pain. It was also a way to bring the family even closer together as all of my siblings and spouses participated in the book in some way.

My siblings, with whom I have been extremely close since childhood. **Jimmy, Marby and Timmy** who have stood by me through the darkest days and the brightest moments even before the dreaded darkness of RSD. They are all successful in their own right and the drive and determination in all we do has kept me on course and not allowed me to give up.

Dr. Mark Rubin, my pain management doctor, from the Arizona Center for Pain Relief in Phoenix, AZ. For being the first doctor to listen to me and put all the pieces together. You were the first doctor I had seen in the last 6 years since the accident who actually took the time to do what would help me. Thank you also for the referral to

Dr. Hummel. You have made my life bearable and I am forever grateful.

Dr. Matthew Hummel, my general practitioner of the Foundation Hills Family Practice in Foundation Hills, AZ. Thank you for working with my pain management doctor to get me the best care available. Your ability to provide excellent care and support has been tremendously helpful in my everyday challenges. I wish everyone a doctor as caring and helpful as you are.

Brett Slavicek, my first friend in Arizona. Thank you for taking me on as a client and helping me fire my first attorney. God put you in my life to serve a major role in helping me, and you came through. You were the first to help me find a purpose after the accident, and you created a job for me when no one else would hire me. When I was at the bottom of my ordeal, your guidance lifted me up. I loved being a legal assistant for you. It taught me new life skills that I could never have learned in my cheerleading career.

John Allison, Dick Eymann and Linda Hansen, thank you for your years of hard work on my case. You were amazing in preparations and in court. You all deserve an award for what you did for me and continue to do for others who have had personal injuries due to someone else's negligence. I am glad that Brett led me to you. I will never forget the fight you lead for me.

Scott K., thank you for helping me find my voice. Because of you, I learned to speak up when things are not right. Learning to take control of my life was one of the greatest gifts I could have been given. Your guidance and life tools help me with living through the pain every day.

Ed Harkins, PT, thank you for helping me through my knee surgery, prior to the RSD and assisting me after the accident that caused the RSD. Because of your care and lessons, I am a stronger person, literally.

Paul Nelson, PT, thank you for all your knowledge on physical therapy with RSD. You are the one who got me on track with what I should and should not be doing and taught me that less activity can be beneficial to my daily health and that it is ok to be open with my healthcare providers.

I would like to acknowledge **Melanie Anne McDowell**, who passed away in 2006. She is my pseudo step- sister (although our parents did not marry, we were raised as family) and my mentor in RSD. Thank you for teaching me about living life with RSD and that I too will be ok. I miss you beyond words and think of you every day. I am sad you are gone but am happy you are no longer suffering with RSD. Also, thanks to the McDowell family for your support even though Melanie and Ralph are no longer with us. (**Anne, Gail and Roni**).

There have been so many others who have helped me along the way. I would not be as well adjusted or supported without you: **Jodi Dragon** for being my best friend and a supporter in this pain fight; **Vance Hudson & Rob Kronenberg** for your support and allowing me the opportunities to speak to others about pain and my experience; the RSDHope staff for choosing me to mentor other patients; **Todd Ellenbecker, PT, & Dr. Ed Tingstad, orthopedic,** for your great medical care and advice. All of the volunteers and board members of the Power of Pain Foundation for their confidence and support of me and RSD awareness- powerofpain.org.

NATIONAL RESOURCES

Power Of Pain Foundation
www.powerofpain.org
804-256-1912

American Chronic Pain Association
www.theacpa.org
1-916-632-0922

American Medical Association
312-464-5000
www.ama-assn.org

American Pain Foundation
www.painfoundation.org
1-888-615-PAIN

American Pain Society
www.ampainsoc.org

Cancer Care
www.cancercare.org
1-800-813-HOPE

Federation of State Medical Boards
817-868-4000
www.fsmb.org

RSDSA
www.rsds.org

POWER OF PAIN FOUNDATION

The Power of Pain Foundation's mission is to educate and show support for chronic pain patients, specifically those with Neuropathy pain conditions including Reflex Sympathetic Dystrophy (RSD), diabetic neuropathy and post cancer pain. Since its inception in

January of 2007, the POPF is dedicated to increasing the number of patients receiving proper care and timely pain relief. We fulfill our mission by promoting public and professional awareness of Neuropathy conditions, educating those afflicted with the syndrome, their families, friends and healthcare providers on the disabling pain and life changes it causes, action-oriented awareness and improve pain care, through activities and efforts to eliminate under treatment and empower patients to be self-advocates, raising funds for financial, emotional and educational support for chronic pain sufferers who have Neuropathy pain conditions and Support research to find a cure for Neuropathy conditions such as RSD.

The foundation objectives are reached by important education, support and enhancement projects that do not receive government funding but are greatly needed. The Power of Pain Foundation demonstrates its commitment to the chronic pain community by promoting new knowledge in the cause and treatment of chronic pain. The Chronic Pain Awareness and Advocacy Program (CPAAP) seeks to accomplish this outcome by providing pain patients, their caretakers, family and healthcare professionals with practical information. The patient's ability to understand healthcare communications including prescription instructions, test results, insurance forms, what to expect as a patient when receiving healthcare, what caretakers can do to assist the pain patient with whom they are working, are addressed in the presentation. Through the CPAAP, we share ideas, build effective strategies, inspire patient action, and unite as a powerful force to improve pain management in our communities and across the nation. We also encourage people with pain to insist on the care they need and deserve, educate people in pain, their families, friends and caretakers about issues surrounding patient rights, pain management and encourage people with pain to demand the care they need and deserve.

The program informs and supports pain patients. We will inform patients by providing up-to-date pain care information, patient rights, and patient responsibilities. We show support through providing resources to people with pain, empower patients to become self-advocates and supply resources to improve care.

The ultimate goal is to allow chronic pain patients the ability to perform their regular activities in the community and to bolster society's ability to provide full opportunities and appropriate supports for its pain citizens.

Through supporting education for pain patients, family members, caretakers and medical professionals, we make an important contribution to the overall knowledge and treatment of chronic pain. This allows our foundation to affect the lives of the millions of people with neuropathy pain nationwide as well as chronic pain patients, caretakers, family members and healthcare professionals.

The Power of Pain Foundation provides community based support services that address the immediate need of Neuropathy pain patients. Grant beneficiaries include patients who are economically and socially affected by these invisible diseases. Whether you have Neuropathy pain or are a caregiver, family member or friend of someone diagnosed, we'll help you face the challenges and life changes of chronic nerve pain, head on.

The POPF coordinates events to raise money for the purpose of education enrichment, leadership-training programs and support projects for chronic pain patients suffering with Neurological conditions. Patients still are not getting a timely diagnosis allowing for proper treatment. More research is needed on these painful diseases. For instance we need so desperately to raise awareness for RSD. The condition of RSD affects both men and woman of all ages and can affect your entire body. Most suffers are affected in the extremities. However, RSD can also attack your eyes, internal organs, and can develop full body. RSD affects females 3 to 1 over men. If a patient is treated in the first 3-9 months of triggering RSD, there is a greater chance of it going into remission. However, after 6-9 months, the remission rate is extremely low. Therefore, education and research are very sorely needed. Most doctors do not study RSD in med school; however, if they knew the signs and symptoms they could save many lives from suffering with this chronic pain nerve disorder.

Foundation programs include: Comic Pain Relief, public service announcements, awareness and advocacy events, internet programs, brochures, diagnostic procedure video distribution, Faces of Motivation, interviews by TV, radio and newspaper outlets, grants for patients and other non-profits, individual patient mentoring and supports, McDowell Pain Advocacy Award, ongoing neuropathy patient and caretaker survey, pain conference vendor, and All I Want for Christmas Campaign. More information on the programs can be found at www.powerofpain.org.

GLOSSARY

Agitation- anxiety, worry, nervousness, tension, distress, to excite and often trouble the mind or feelings of

Allodynia- pain resulting from a stimulus (as a light touch of the skin) which would not normally provoke pain

Anticonvulsants- Antiepileptic drugs are medicines that reduce convulsions

Antidepressants- used or tending to relieve or prevent psychic depression

Anxiety- nervousness or agitation, often about something that is going to happen, PSYCHIATRY a medical condition marked by intense apprehension or fear of real or imagined danger

Arthroscopy- Invasive procedure involving the inspection of the inside of a joint of the body using an endoscope- a medical instrument consisting of a long tube inserted into the body, used for diagnostic examination and surgical procedures

Atrophy- decrease in size or wasting away of a body part or tissue; loss of a part or organ incidental to the normal development of life

Automatic Inflammation Response- local response to cellular injury that is marked by capillary dilatation, leukocytic infiltration, redness, heat, pain, swelling, and often loss of function and that serves as a mechanism initiating the elimination of noxious agents and of damaged tissue

Autonomic Nervous System (ANS)- a part of the vertebrate nervous system that innervates smooth and cardiac muscle and glandular tissues and governs involuntary actions (as secretion, vasoconstriction, or peristalsis) and that consists of the sympathetic nervous system and the parasympathetic nervous system -- called also vegetative nervous system

Biofeedback- the technique of making unconscious or involuntary bodily processes (as heartbeat or brain waves) perceptible to the senses (as by the use of an oscilloscope) in order to manipulate them by conscious mental control

Blood Flow- the movement of blood through the vessels of the body that is induced by the pumping action of the heart and serves to distribute nutrients and oxygen to and remove waste products from all parts of the body

Board Certification- Board certified doctors are required to have extra training after medical school to become specialists in a particular field of medicine and are required to take continuing education courses in order to maintain their board certification status

Body Fatigue- the temporary loss of power to respond induced in a sensory receptor or motor end organ by continued stimulation

Body Scan 3-D- to examine especially systematically with a sensing device (as a photometer or a beam of radiation)

Brachial Plexus- a complex network of nerves that is formed chiefly by the lower four cervical nerves and the first thoracic nerve, lies partly within the axilla, and supplies nerves to the chest, shoulder, and arm

Bursitis- inflammation of a bursa (as of the shoulder or elbow)

Cancer- a malignant tumor of potentially unlimited growth that expands locally by invasion and systemically by metastasis

Cardiovascular Condition- of, relating to, or involving the heart and blood vessels: cardiovascular disease

Carpal Tunnel Syndrome- a condition caused by compression of the median nerve in the carpal tunnel and characterized especially by weakness, pain, and disturbances of sensation in the hand and fingers

Causalgia- a persistent burning sensation of the skin, caused usually by injury to a peripheral nerve

Cellulites- deposits of subcutaneous fat within fibrous connective tissue (as in the thighs, hips, and buttocks) that give a puckered and dimpled appearance to the skin surface

Central Nerve System- the part of the nervous system, consisting of the brain and spinal cord, which controls and coordinates most functions of the body and mind. Impulses from sense organs travel to the central nervous system and impulses to muscles and glands travel from it

Chronic Diseases- describes an illness or medical condition that lasts over a long period and sometimes causes a long-term change in the body

Clinical history- a record of signs and symptoms of an individual's personal/family history & environment for use in analysis or instructive illustration

Complications- a secondary disease or condition that develops in the course of a primary disease or condition and arises either because of it or from independent causes

Corticosteroids- any of various adrenal-cortex steroids (as corticosterone, cortisone, and aldosterone) that are divided based on their major biological activity into glucocorticoids and mineralocorticoids

Cure- a medication or treatment that brings about a full recovery from an illness or injury

Depression- an act of depressing or a state of being depressed: as a (1): a state of feeling sad (2): a psychoneurotic or psychotic disorder marked especially by sadness, inactivity, difficulty with thinking and concentration, a significant increase or decrease in appetite and time spent sleeping, feelings of dejection and hopelessness, and sometimes suicidal thoughts or an attempt to commit suicide b: a reduction in functional activity, amount, quality, or force

Diabetic Neuropathy- degenerative state of the nervous system or nerves; a systemic condition that stems from a neuropathy of or relating to diabetes

Disk Hernia- a protrusion of a part through connective
tissue, which it is normally enclosed

Doctor- health services a title used before the names of
health professionals such as dentists, veterinarians, and
osteopaths, health services somebody qualified and
licensed to give people medical treatment, education a title
given to somebody who has been awarded a doctorate, the
highest level of degree awarded by a university

Dry Mouth Syndrome- Dry mouth is a common side
effect of many prescription and nonprescription drugs,
including drugs used to treat depression, anxiety, pain,
allergies and colds, obesity, acne, epilepsy, hypertension,
diarrhea, nausea, psychotic disorders, urinary incontinence,
asthma and Parkinson's disease. Dry mouth is also a side
effect of muscle relaxants and sedatives. Dry mouth can be
a result of nerve damage to the head and neck area from an
injury or surgery. Common symptoms of dry mouth
include: A sticky, dry feeling in the mouth, Frequent thirst,
Sores in the mouth; sores or split skin at the corners of the
mouth; cracked lips, A dry feeling in the throat, A burning

or tingling sensation in the mouth and especially on the tongue, A dry, red, raw tongue, Problems speaking or difficulty tasting, chewing and swallowing, Hoarseness, dry nasal passages, sore throat

Dystonia Edema- swelling of a limb, a neurological disorder that causes involuntary muscle spasms and twisting of the limbs

Dystrophy- progressive degeneration of a body tissue such as muscle, caused by inadequate nourishment of the affected part, as a result of some known or unknown cause

Edema- a buildup of excess serous fluid between tissue cells

EMG- electromyogram, graphical tracing of the electrical activity in a muscle at rest or during contraction, used to diagnose nerve and muscle disorders

Emotional Disturbances- a conscious mental reaction (as anger or fear) subjectively experienced as strong feeling usually directed toward a specific object and typically accompanied by physiological and behavioral changes in the body

Explanation of Benefits (EOB)- Explanation of Benefit forms (EOB's) are sent by payers to both enrollees and providers. EOB's provide necessary information about claim payment information and patient responsibility amounts.

FDA - the federal agency that oversees trade in and the safety of food and drugs in the United States

Fever- a rise of body temperature above the normal whether a natural response (as to infection) or artificially induced for therapeutic reasons, an abnormal bodily state characterized by increased production of heat, accelerated heart action and pulse, and systemic debility with weakness, loss of appetite, and thirst

First Rib Resection- the surgical removal of the first rib

Fluoride- a chemical compound consisting of fluorine and another element or group

Functional MRI- magnetic resonance imaging used to demonstrate correlations between physical changes (as in blood flow) in the brain and mental functioning (as in performing cognitive tasks)

Ganglion Nerve Bundle- a mass of nerve tissue containing cell bodies of neurons that is located outside the central nervous system and forms an enlargement upon a nerve or upon two or more nerves at their point of junction or separation

Gastrointestinal- relating to the stomach and intestines

General Doctor- a doctor regularly consulted by a family in time of medical need

Gout- metabolic disease marked by a painful inflammation of the joints, deposits of urates in and around the joints, and usually an excessive amount of uric acid in the blood

Guilt- an awareness of having done wrong or committed a crime, accompanied by feelings of shame and regret

Health Insurance- an arrangement by which a company gives customers financial protection against loss or harm such as theft or illness in return for payment premium.

HMO- A health maintenance organization (HMO) is a type of managed care organization (MCO) that provides a form of health care coverage in the United States that is fulfilled through hospitals, doctors, and other providers with which the HMO has a contract. The Health Maintenance Organization Act of 1973 required employers with 25 or more employees to offer federally certified HMO options. Unlike traditional indemnity insurance, an HMO covers only care rendered by those doctors and other professionals who have agreed to treat patients in accordance with the HMO's guidelines and restrictions in exchange for a steady stream of customers.

PPO- A preferred provider organization is a managed care organization of medical doctors, hospitals, and other health care providers who have covenanted with an insurer or a third-party administrator to provide health care at reduced rates to the insurer's or administrator's clients. The idea of a preferred provider organization is that the providers will provide the insured members of the group a substantial discount below their regularly charged rates. This will be mutually beneficial in theory, as the insurer will be billed at a reduced rate when its insured utilize the services of the "preferred" provider and the provider will see an increase in its business as almost all insured people in the organization will use only providers who are members. Even the insured should benefit, as lower costs to the insurer should result in lower rates of increase in premiums. Preferred provider organizations themselves earn money by charging an access fee to the insurance company for the use of their network. They negotiate with providers to set fee schedules, and handle disputes between insurers and providers. PPOs can also contract with one another to strengthen their position in certain geographic areas without forming new relationships directly with providers. Under the PPO, you would simply pay more for going to a non-preferred provider.

EPO- An exclusive provider organization (EPO), is similar to a PPO, but if you seek care from a non-preferred provider you will not receive any coverage at all, unless there is a state mandate preventing the plan from differentiating between preferred and non-preferred provider. EPOs are less common than PPOs.

Health Insurance Coverage- insurance against loss through illness of the insured, insurance providing compensation for medical expenses

Hearing- the act or power of apprehending sound; specifically: one of the special senses of vertebrates that is concerned with the perception of sound, is mediated through the organ of Corti of the ear in mammals, is normally sensitive in humans to sound vibrations between 16 and 27,000 hertz but most receptive to those between 2000 and 5000 hertz, is conducted centrally by the cochlear branch of the auditory nerve, and is coordinated especially in the medial geniculate body

Horner's Syndrome- a syndrome marked by sinking in of the eyeball, contraction of the pupil, drooping of the upper eyelid, and vasodilatation and anhidrosis of the face, and caused by paralysis of the cervical sympathetic nerve fibers on the affected side

Hydrotherapy- the treatment of injuries and physical conditions by a trained person under the supervision of a specialist in physical medicine performed in water

Hyperalgesia- overly painful response to a minimal stimulus

Hypersensitive- excessively or abnormally sensitive

Immobilization- medicine to rest a joint or keep the parts of a fractured limb fixed in place so that they are unable to move

Immune System- the bodily system that protects the body from foreign substances, cells, and tissues by producing the immune response and that includes especially the thymus, spleen, lymph nodes, special deposits of lymphoid tissue (as in the gastrointestinal tract and bone marrow), lymphocytes including the B cells and T cells, and antibodies

Inflammation Response- swelling, redness, heat, and pain produced in an area of the body as a reaction to injury or infection, Inflammation (Latin, inflammation, to set on fire) is the complex biological response of vascular tissues to harmful stimuli, such as pathogens, damaged cells, or irritants. It is a protective attempt by the organism to remove the injurious stimuli as well as initiate the healing process for the tissue. In the absence of inflammation, wounds and infections would never heal and progressive destruction of the tissue would compromise the survival of the organism. However, inflammation that runs unchecked can also lead to a host of diseases; it is for this reason that inflammation is normally tightly regulated by the body. Inflammation can be classified as either acute or chronic. Acute inflammation is the initial response of the body to harmful stimuli and is achieved by the increased movement of plasma and leukocytes from the blood into the injured tissues. A cascade of biochemical events propagates and matures the inflammatory response, involving the local vascular system, the immune system, and various cells within the injured tissue. Prolonged inflammation, known as chronic inflammation, leads to a progressive shift in the type of cells which are present at the site of inflammation and is characterized by simultaneous destruction and healing of the tissue from the inflammatory process

Infusion- medicine the introduction of a solution such as Ketamine, Lidocaine, saline, sucrose, or glucose through a drip feed in order to treat or feed a patient

Injury Rehabilitation- Injury rehabilitation protocols are commonly used after a serious sports injury or post-surgery and are an important part of recovery. These protocols often include specific strength and flexibility exercises to help build strength and range of motion in an injured extremity

Intrathecal- something that happens inside the spinal canal. An Intrathecal injection, as in a spinal anaesthesia or in chemotherapy or pain management applications. This route is also used for some infections, particularly post-neurosurgical. The drug needs to be given this way to avoid the blood brain barrier. The same drug given orally must enter the blood stream and has a much harder time reaching the brain; by the time it does, most of the drug has been absorbed by the body's system and is excreted

Intrathecal Pump- An Intrathecal pump is a medical device used to deliver very small quantities of medications directly to the spinal fluid of a human being. Medications such as Baclofen, morphine, or Ziconotide may be delivered in this manner to minimize the side effects often associated with the higher dosages commonly found in oral medications of the same type

Invasive Procedure- A medical procedure that invades (enters) the body, usually by cutting or puncturing the skin or by inserting instruments into the body

Invisible Disability- inability to pursue an occupation because of physical or mental impairment due to a condition that is not readily apparent to other people

Irritability- the property of protoplasm and of living organisms that permits them to react to stimuli, extremely sensitive, especially to inflammation

Isokinetic Testing- Isokinetic testing is performed with a constant speed of angular motion but variable resistance. Isokinetic dynamometers have been shown to produce relatively reliable data when testing. Isokinetic testing can be helpful during the rehabilitation of orthopedic patients, since it allows easy monitoring of progress. It also enables the patient to work on muscle rehabilitation in a controlled manner at higher speeds than are possible with more conventional exercise equipment

IV (intravenous)- the equipment used to administer an IV, the injection of quantities of a therapeutic fluid such as blood, plasma, saline, or glucose directly into somebody's vein at an adjustable rate

Limbic System- a group of sub cortical structures (as the hypothalamus, the hippocampus, and the amygdala) of the brain that are concerned especially with emotion and motivation

Lymphedema- a form of edema resulting from the loss of normal lymph channel drainage of the affected part Lymph vessels may be blocked by cancer or by parasitic filarial worms, or may have been removed in the course of cancer surgery

Malingering- to pretend to be ill, especially in order to avoid work

Meniscus- a fibrous cartilage within a joint, either, of two crescent-shaped lamellae of fibrocartilage that border and partly cover the articulating surfaces of the tibia and femur at the knee

Migraines- condition that is marked by a recurrent, usually unilateral severe headache many times accompanied by nausea, vomiting and followed by sleep, that tends to occur in more than one member of a family, and that is of uncertain origin though attacks appear to be precipitated by dilatation of intracranial blood vessels

MRA- magnetic resonance imaging used to visualize noninvasively the heart, blood vessels, or blood flow in the circulatory system -- abbreviation MRA; called also MR angiography

MRI- an imaging technique that uses electromagnetic radiation to obtain images of the body's soft tissues, e.g. the brain and spinal cord the body is subjected to a powerful magnetic field, allowing tiny signals from atomic nuclei to be detected and then processed and converted into images by a computer. Is used to demonstrate correlations between physical changes (as in blood flow) in the brain and mental functioning (as in performing cognitive tasks)

Narcotic Analgesics- drug which causes insensibility to pain without loss of consciousness, that in moderate doses dulls the senses, relieves pain, and induces profound sleep but in excessive doses causes stupor, coma, or convulsions

Neoplasm- a new growth of tissue serving no physiological function

Nerves- any of the filamentous bands of nervous tissue that connect parts of the nervous system with the other organs, conduct nervous impulses, and are made up of axons and dendrites together with protective and supportive structures and that for the larger nerves have the fibers gathered into funiculi surrounded by a perineurium and the funiculi enclosed in a common epineurium

Nerve Bundle- a bundle of fibers forming a network that transmits messages in the form of impulses between the brain or spinal cord and the body's organs Motor nerves carry impulses outward to the muscles and glands, while sensory nerves carry inbound information about the body's movements and sensations. Mixed nerves perform both functions

Nerve entrapment- chronic compression of a peripheral nerve (as the median nerve or ulnar nerve) usually between ligamentous and bony surfaces that is characterized especially by pain, numbness, tingling, or weakness

Nervous System- a large system of nerves, the network of nerve cells and nerve fibers in most animals that conveys sensations to the brain and motor impulses to organs and muscles

Neurological Condition- a branch of medicine concerned especially with the structure, functions, and diseases of the nervous system

Neurologist- a person specializing in neurology, a physician skilled in the diagnosis and treatment of disease of the nervous system

Neurons- one of the cells that constitute nervous tissue, that have the property of transmitting and receiving nervous impulses, and that are composed of somewhat reddish or grayish protoplasm with a large nucleus containing a conspicuous nucleolus, irregular cytoplasmic granules, and cytoplasmic processes which are highly differentiated frequently as multiple dendrites or usually as solitary axons and which conduct impulses toward and away from the nerve cell body

Neuropathy- a disease or disorder, especially a degenerative one, which affects the nervous system

Non-invasive Procedure- not tending to infiltrate and destroy healthy tissue, not being or involving an invasive medical procedure, noninvasive imaging techniques that do not require the injection of dyes

Nuclear Bone Scans- chemical analysis that uses nuclear magnetic resonance especially to study molecular structure

Obsessive Compulsive Disorder- a psychoneurotic disorder in which the patient is beset with obsessions or compulsions or both and suffers extreme anxiety or depression through failure to think the obsessive thoughts or perform the compelling acts -- abbreviation OCD; called also obsessive-compulsive neurosis, obsessive-compulsive reaction

Occupational Therapy/OT- therapy based on engagement in meaningful activities of daily life (as self-care skills, education, work, or social interaction) especially to enable or encourage participation in such activities despite impairments or limitations in physical or mental functioning

Oral Opioids- a synthetic drug (as methadone) possessing narcotic properties similar to opiates but not derived from opium taken by mouth

Orthopedic- the branch of medicine concerned with the nature and correction of disorders of the bones, joints, ligaments, or muscles

Osteoarthritis- arthritis typically with onset during middle or old age that is characterized by degenerative and sometimes hypertrophic changes in the bone and cartilage of one or more joints and a progressive wearing down of apposing joint surfaces with consequent distortion of joint position and is marked symptomatically especially by pain, swelling, and stiffness -- abbreviation OA

Osteomyelitis/Bone Infection– infectious usually painful inflammatory disease of bone that is often of bacterial origin and may result in death of bone tissue

Osteoporosis- a condition that affects especially older women and is characterized by decrease in bone mass with decreased density and enlargement of bone spaces producing porosity and brittleness

Pain- a basic bodily sensation that is induced by a noxious stimulus, is received by naked nerve endings, is characterized by physical discomfort (as pricking, throbbing, or aching), and typically leads to evasive action

> **Acute-** lasting a short period of time, typically less than 6 months, ending when the injury is healed
> **Chronic-** a state of physical, emotional, or mental lack of well-being or physical, emotional, or mental uneasiness that lasts more than the appropriate healing time for the injury/insult

Pain Clinic- These centers are called by many different names, including: pain clinic, pain management center, pain center, pain unit or pain service. These facilities may be in a wing of your local hospital or medical center, in a separate medical-professional building or in a doctor's office. Some are affiliated with medical schools and large health care centers

Patella- a flat triangular bone located at the front of the knee. It protects the knee joint, also known as a kneecap

Periodontal Disease- Periodontal disease is an infection of the tissues that support your teeth. Periodontal diseases attack just below the gum line in the sulcus, where they cause the attachment of the tooth and its supporting tissues to break down. As the tissues are damaged, the sulcus develops into a pocket: generally, the more severe the disease, the greater the depth of the pocket

Peripheral Neuropathy- a disease or degenerative state (as polyneuropathy) of the peripheral nerves in which motor, sensory, or vasomotor nerve fibers may be affected and which is marked by muscle weakness and atrophy, pain, and numbness

Physical Therapy- the treatment of disease by physical and mechanical means (as massage, regulated exercise, water, light, heat, and electricity)

Physiotherapy- the treatment of injuries and physical conditions by a trained person under the supervision of a specialist in physical medicine

Procedure- any means of doing or accomplishing something

Prognosis- the prospect of survival and recovery from a disease as anticipated from the usual course of that disease or indicated by special features of the case

Psychologist- a specialist in one or more branches of psychology, a practitioner of clinical psychology, counseling, or guidance

Radiofrequency Ablation- procedure that uses radio-frequency heat to collapse veins

Recovery- the act of regaining or returning toward a normal or healthy state

Reflexes- automatic and often inborn response to a stimulus that involves a nerve impulse passing inward from a receptor to the spinal cord and thence outward to an effector (as a muscle or gland) without reaching the level of consciousness and often without passing to the brain

REM (rapid eye movement)- a rapid conjugate movement of the eyes associated especially with REM sleep

Remission- a state or period during which the symptoms of a disease are abated

Resentment- aggrieved feelings caused by a sense of having been badly treated

Rheumatoid Arthritis- a usually chronic disease that is considered an autoimmune disease and is characterized especially by pain, stiffness, inflammation, swelling, and sometimes destruction of joints -- abbreviation RA; called also atrophic arthritis

Septic Arthritis- Infectious arthritis is caused by a germ that travels through the body to a joint. The germ can be a bacterium, virus, or fungus. The germ can enter the body though the skin, nose, throat, ears, or through an open wound. Most often, infectious arthritis develops after an existing infection anywhere in the body travels through the bloodstream to a joint

Short-term Memory Problems- loss of memory that involves recall of information for a relatively short time

Skin Rashes- an eruption on the body typically with little or no elevation above the surface

Sleep Disorder/Insomnia- prolonged and usually abnormal inability to obtain adequate sleep -- called also agrypnia

Small Nerve Biopsy- the removal and examination of small nerve tissue from the living body

Small-fiber Degeneration- Small fiber neuropathy is a relatively common disorder often associated with systemic conditions, such as diabetes, HIV, and vasculitis. Painful burning feet with diminished pain and temperature perception, and in some cases autonomic dysfunction, characterize this syndrome. Despite the magnitude of the symptoms, there are few objective measures to identify and quantify these neuropathies

Spasms- an involuntary and abnormal contraction of muscle or muscle fibers or of a hollow organ (as an artery, the colon, or the esophagus) that consists largely of involuntary muscle fiber

Spinal Cord Stimulator- Spinal cord stimulation (SCS) is an implantable device that uses an electrical current to treat chronic pain. A small pulse generator, implanted in the back, transmits electrical pulses to the spinal cord. These pulses interfere with the nerve impulses

Stress- mental, emotional, or physical strain caused by anxiety or overwork, It may cause such symptoms as raised blood pressure or depression

Sudomotor Activity- of, relating to, or being nerve fibers controlling the activity of sweat glands, increase or decrease of perspiration

Surgeon- a medical specialist who performs surgery: a physician qualified to treat those diseases that are amenable to or require surgery

Surgery- a branch of medicine concerned with diseases and conditions requiring or amenable to operative or manual procedures

Surgical Procedures- surgery involving a risk to the life of the patient, an operation upon an organ within the cranium, chest, abdomen, or pelvic cavity

Sweating- the clear salty liquid that passes to the surface of the skin when somebody is hot or as a result of strenuous activity, fear, anxiety, or illness

Swelling- an increase in size of part of the body, typically because of injury, infection, or other medical condition

Sympathectomy- refers to the destruction of tissue anywhere in either of the two sympathetic trunks, long chains of nerve ganglia lying along either side of the spine.

Each trunk is broadly divided into three regions: cervical (up by the neck), thoracic (in the chest) and lumbar (lower back). The most common area targeted in Sympathectomy is the upper thoracic region, that part of the sympathetic chain lying between the first and fifth thoracic vertebrae

Sympathetic Nerve Block- an interruption of the passage of impulses through a nerve (as with pressure or narcotization)

Sympathetic Nervous System (SNS)- the part of the autonomic nervous system that is concerned especially with preparing the body to react to situations of stress or emergency, that contains chiefly adrenergic fibers and tends to depress secretion, decrease the tone and contractility of smooth muscle, increase heart rate, and that consists essentially of preganglionic fibers arising in the thoracic and upper lumbar parts of the spinal cord and passing through delicate white rami communicantes to ganglia located in a pair of sympathetic chains situated one on each side of the spinal column or to more peripheral ganglia or ganglionated plexuses and postganglionic fibers passing typically through gray rami communicantes to spinal nerves with which they are distributed to various end organs -- called also sympathetic system

Sympathetically Independent Pain (SIP)- when the pain becomes centrally maintained only (there are now changes in the nerve cells in the spinal cord), and sympathetic blocks have little or no effect on it whatsoever

Sympathetically Maintained Pain (SMP)- patients can present with any of the symptoms of RSD on their own. They can present with just swelling, just Allodynia, just burning pain, muscle spasm, etc., and if these people respond to sympathetic blocks, they are then defined as having sympathetically maintained pain

Symptoms- subjective evidence of disease or physical disturbance observed by the patient, something that indicates the presence of a physical disorder

Syndrome- a group of signs and symptoms that together is characteristic or indicative of a specific disease or other disorder

Tendonitis- inflammation of a tendon

Tens Unit- Sticky patches (electrodes) are attached to the skin, and small electrical impulses are delivered to underlying nerve fibers. This works in two ways. The first is through endorphins. The body has its own mechanisms for suppressing pain. It releases natural chemicals called endorphins in the brain, which act as pain relieving substances. TENS units can activate this mechanism. Secondly, the electrical stimulation of the nerve fibers through the electrodes can actually block a pain signal from being carried all the way to the brain. If it is blocked, the pain is not felt

Thermogram- technique for detecting and measuring variations in the heat emitted by various regions of the body and transforming them into visible signals that can be recorded photographically

Thoracic Outlet Syndrome- For the most part, these disorders are produced by compression of the components of the brachial plexus (the large cluster of nerves that pass from the neck to the arm), the subclavian artery, or the subclavian vein. These subtypes are referred to as Neurogenic TOS, arterial TOS, and venous TOS, respectively. The Neurogenic form of TOS accounts for 95 to 98% of all cases of TOS

Tinnitus- a sensation of noise (as a ringing or roaring) that is caused by a bodily condition (as a disturbance of the auditory nerve or wax in the ear) and typically is of the subjective form that can only be heard by the one affected

TMJ Syndrome- Temporomandibular joint syndrome is a medical problem related to the jaw joint. The TMJ connects the lower jaw (mandible) to the skull (temporal bone) in front of the ear. Problems in this area can cause head and neck pain, a jaw that is locked in position or difficult to open, problems biting, and popping sounds when you bite

Traction- the application of a pulling force for medical purposes, e.g. to reduce a fracture, maintain bone alignment, relieve pain, or prevent spinal injury

Trauma- an injury to living tissue caused by an extrinsic agent

Tremors- a trembling or shaking usually from physical weakness, emotional stress, or disease

Vascular Study- a noninvasive (the skin is not pierced) procedure used to assess the blood flow in arteries and veins. A transducer (like a microphone) sends out ultrasonic sound waves at a frequency too high to be heard. When the transducer is placed on the skin at certain locations and angles, the ultrasonic sound waves move through the skin and other body tissues to the blood vessels, where the waves echo off the blood cells. The transducer picks up the reflected waves and sends them to an amplifier, which makes the ultrasonic sound waves audible.

Vision- the special sense by which the qualities of an object (as color, luminosity, shape, and size) constituting its appearance are perceived through a process in which light rays entering the eye are transformed by the retina into electrical signals that are transmitted to the brain via the optic nerve

Whiplash- injury resulting from a sudden sharp whipping movement of the neck and head (as of a person in a vehicle that is struck head-on or from the rear by another vehicle)

X-Rays- any of the electromagnetic radiations of the same nature as visible radiation but of an extremely short wavelength less than 100 angstroms that is produced by bombarding a metallic target with fast electrons in vacuum or by transition of atoms to lower energy states and that has the properties of ionizing a gas upon passage through it, of penetrating various thicknesses of all solids, of producing secondary radiations by impinging on material bodies, of acting on photographic films and plates as light does, and of causing fluorescent screens to emit light -- called also roentgen ray

OTHER INGLE BOOKS

ReMission Possible; Yours If You Choose To Accept It

The Pain Code; A Patient Journal For Better
Communication With Their Healthcare Professionals
(Supplement To RSD In Me!)

The Wisdom of Ingle;
Fall Down And Get Up In Half A Day

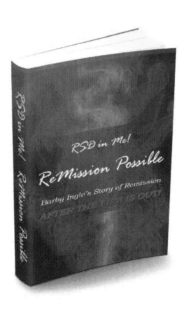